Health over Harmony

Originally published by:
East-West Publishing

Paul Sweeney
C/O East-West Publishing
P.O. Box 308
Scottsdale AZ 85252.
healthoverharmony@gmail.com
healthoverharmony.com

Health over Harmony 501c Phx AZ (Contributions Appreciated)

ALL RAW FOOD REFERENCES REFER TO ORGANIC OR NATURALLY GROWN FOODS

Printed in the United States of America and

Japan Copyright © 2008-2019 Paul Sweeney

ISBN: 9798655926134

(Vol 1 ISBN 13: 9781439259504)

Health over Harmony

Healing techniques and 2020 technology for coming pandemics

Paul Sweeney Acup. Physician

Lic. Acup. Certified in Mental Health

(Certified Uechi-ryu Instructor)

Edited by Dr Ann Cauble

OUTLINE (as Table of Contents)

- toxicity of all cooked carbohydrates and advanced glycation end- products and cross-linking of molecules
- acrylamides
- toxicity of non-organic meat/farm fish and "mad cow"
- benefits of raw meats in healing
- heterocyclic amines and lipid oxides from cooked proteins and fat
- the significance of raw fats being able to rebuild the nervous system, draw out heavy metals and strip cooked fat deposits from tissues
- **simple powerful aerobic bacterial ingestion for true healing and detoxification;** how I dispel erroneous fears associated with raw meats and bacteria ingestion, how I both encourage patients and friends to use and I personally use raw foods and bacteria daily.
- **my first raw dairy experience in Spain** with the gypsies (raw goat milk and blood mixture given to me to heal my illness)
- my first experience with Japanese poisonous "tora-hugu"
- **the strong hold that the consensus reality has on people** and the psychological **shift necessary to heal (truth over harmony)**
- science versus fear (truth over harmony)
- bacteria as a living race and future probiotics
- hospitals testing viruses for cancer cures

Development of Human Consciousness through the Human Organs

- Chinese basic medical/philosophical theory and the 12 organ pairing

- "The very process of evolution is determined, in part, by how people, as enlightened humans, consciously choose to understand, develop and manifest the spiritual energies inherent in each organ."

- how one connects to the significance of one's organs initially through illness or pain and the healing path made available and usually ignored by illness and pain.,
- rejection of underlying significance of symbolic connections and the animal-self
- various forms of consciousness and the development of emotional consciousness and emotional intelligence

- "The point is to allow consciousness itself to develop in several different ways as if to involve emotional and animal consciousness leading at the deeper level to the understanding and awareness that comes from the organs themselves; as if recognizing their innate intelligence."

Section II: Heart/ Small Intestine Example

- I use the poignant example of the small intestine/ heart yin-yang pairing to elucidate the emotional/ physiological significance of the organs on a practical and clinical level.

• why the small intestine/heart pairing is so significant for humanity at the present time

• examples of the heart's physiological manifestation of lacking small intestine absorptive qualities such as heart murmur, arrhythmia, size, circulatory function and insulin problems.
• examples of the small intestine's physiological manifestation of lacking heart love capabilities as a way in which self-love and the ability to receive support from the environment .

• discussion of the Chinese process of treating the small intestine to treat spinal problems: the role of calcium, manganese and bacterial interaction in the small intestine in healing
• connection between depression and depleted bacterial counts in the small intestine
• arthritis as a cleaning mechanism for the body
• brain/small intestine balancing and bacterial intelligence
• genetic incompletion and theory of new meridians forming that have not yet been brought into human DNA (and its implications)

Chapter 8: CASE STUDIES   119

• Succinct informative cases and healing approaches that can offer the reader a new approach to looking at common problems in life outside of the specific medical imbalance highlighted in each case.

• energetic/spiritual/psychological aspects of each case and how these relate to the physical imbalance. A general treatment plan including raw foods, psychological shifts needed by each patient and progress or failure are discussed.

• considering the good point of any imbalance • raw foods, magnesium and calcium impaction on the nerves

Case 6: Pregnancy/ RAW toddler diet

• "The child will eventually learn that his own higher subtle bodies can be used for his own healing, his own strengthening and do not have to be pulled into areas that the parents are unconsciously attracted to. The mother had to pay attention to what she was worrying about all day long, as these energies would be telling the child that one draws one's energy from others, from outside sources, from affairs of the world; this is not true."

• meditation as an aid in treatment insight
• sometimes relieving the patient's main complaint first often adds credibility to the clinician's words and the patient can then open their mind to other ideas
• unacknowledged personal addictions.
• intuitive awakening and spiritual readings to reawaken positive energies that were shut down as a child
• **psychological approach to nurturing a foundation for a raw toddler diet**
• meditation to quicken the resonance between mother and child
• vaccine toxicity and mutated viruses and antibodies
• homeopathic nosodes made from live virus pustules as the only safe real means to confer immunity to a live virus.
• watching the baby/child's reaction to medicine and chemicals

Chapter Nine: Vibrational Treatments

- Homeopathy (microbial, gems, minerals, flowers)
- subtle body treatment
- utilizing the Earth's Schumann resonance to heal

- "For some people any frequency or subtle energy technique will be insufficient for healing because they need more physicalized treatment that can not be brought by subtle energy alone."

- the complexity of the human frequencies and realistic adjustments
- wave forms and electrical stimulation connections
- organ entrainment through frequency
- the reflex pattern and superior healing potential of voice
- **APPENDICES:**
- **Low Deuterium Water**
- **105F Detox Bath and Lymph Issues**
- **Inert Gas Healing**
- **Scalar, Tesla Coil, Frequencies & inert gases**
- **Starting the Raw Diet Basics**
- **Healing by Nature**
- **Reality over Illusion-self healing is inherent**

PREFACE

In this book I am sharing some insights and knowledge with respect to clinically applied energetics, psychology and healing based on 30 years of international travel, clinical work, formal spiritual and Martial Art training in Europe, Africa, North America and Asia. I believe human nature strives to be happy. Therefore, this book's appeal rests on the offering of a fresh positive perspective of life and healing that has led many to find an increased sense of joy in their lives. People are more and more willing and capable of seeing their lives from a new perspective even if doing so goes against the established mass consciousness. People are choosing truth over harmony in their lives.

I mentally relive many emotions in my life: the magic of being lost in contemplation of the night stars from an isolated tropical South China Sea island; the fear of being in a Moroccan holding cell; my despair over the tragic lives and deaths of friends and patients. However, in writing this book, I chose to concentrate on the more important ideas that culminated from these experiences as opposed to stressing the exotic experiences themselves.

I have had the good fortune of traveling afar and learning from many disciples of various schools of thought. Many people exert much time and effort debating the superiority of one philosophy, theory, or sensei over another. Many well-respected gurus, monks, doctors, healers have acquired reputations involving exotic mysterious and hard to believe deeds and ancestral lineage. I feel strongly that if one gains value from anyone regardless of what he would claim as his identity or experience, then perhaps, value remains and one can do something with it. This perspective, on the other hand, will inherently create limitations which naturally occur when one names anything, defines it, and limits it. These limitations then stand in the way of the next step of where the energy and information is used. It is simply a matter then of determining in which areas it would be limiting.

Many things in this book are serious and heavy but it is very important to remember to also have fun with these ideas and techniques as they can lead to health, increased strength physically and mentally and a sense of joy and purpose.

Love dissolves all Karma

In the 2020s, the human species most likely path will be further degradation. The hope of human healing is using low deuterium water, Inert Gases and Scalar-Wave based technology. These should heal millions. They should also help protect us from the toxic Brillouin-Precursors produced by 5G microwave radiation above 24 Gigahertz. This amazing technology is now available and healing thousands to prepare them for the next step in human evolution i.e., a microbiological pandemic. Pandemics force us to work together, empathize, prioritize and evolve emotionally as well as genetically via microbial DNA becoming part of human DNA. **Humans must evolve or or go back to the bad normal and degenerate.**

These advanced amazing healing tools, depending on how they are designed and used are able to both alter our biology physically, as well as, in a different mode, also allow for subtle body (etheric, astral, causal etc) integration which is one definition of human evolution. As humans use these advanced tools, they will be able to do things that used to be, practically speaking, impossible and evolve rapidly. These gifts to humanity are necessary now as the Earth is at a critical junction which could go either way i.e., evolution or destruction. The status quo can not continue.

Humans must look outside their selfish limited "world" of family and friends to include their country, the planet and finally the universal energies to allow us to integrate fully.

The 2020s will be a major evaluation point for the Earth and thus human existence in the near future with coming pandemics which will seem terrible but are the way that many humans will graduate to the next energetic level of love and community. Research suggests that 5G microwaves from over 50,000 satellites will undermine human health and predispose humans to microbial pandemics more and more. Still, humans choose to evolve or devolve with every choice !

It must be understood that microbes clean us and the human immune system kills us as it overreacts to the cleaning of the microbe (bacteria, viral, and parasitic). Natural microbes that have manipulated by man kill quickly -as in HIV and Ebola (and others to come). Microbes like virus, bacteria and parasites are special in that they speed up human and animal physical evolution by directly adding to human DNA (**about 8% of human DNA is viral in nature**). Survivors will be more fit evolutionary wise. **We still have no vaccines for HIV**, Dengue, CMV, RSV and Chikungunya so don't wait on one!

Using some of the ideas and science in this book many will be able to evolve and heal/detox enough so they can , in sufficient numbers withstand the purifying/ cleansing/ detoxifying effects of virus and bacteria alike in the coming pandemics. Microbes evolved to clean us and make humans perfect host for them- a synergistic relationship not well understood. To consciously connect with these entities will allow for rapid healing and evolution. **Viruses and bacteria are the greatest doctors/healers on this planet.** It is the human immune system which overacts to cleansing microbes which kills humans via inflammation, fevers and cellular destruction (well-known cytokine storm events). Hence bats carry many deadly diseases but their immune system doesn't overreact to them so the bats don't "get sick. "

Any microbe that kills quickly as in HIV, Ebola, SARS and even Covid19 has logically been altered by humans for various purposes. When a virus like the hemorrhagic Ebola circulates, even a weakened form that we see now in Africa in 2017, we will tragically see how this recent corona strain is comparatively very mild. Ebola used to kill 100% of infected quickly so it couldn't spread as much as everyone would die before they could spread it from village to village. Now mutations have made it maybe only 50% fatal so it will be able to spread and could kill 100s of millions as is. Ebola vaccines have failed. Ebola is awful as it causes systemic internal bleeding. **Some viruses mutate too fast for a vaccine.**

The only scientific way to prepare for coming pandemics is to detox the body enough so that the microbe will have little reaction in our body (as we see with annual Influenza , Rhino and Corona viruses infecting 100s of millions with little to no symptoms thus not triggering the lethal immune response we see in the many elderly who do die.). Through techniques in this book humans can detox the many cooked food mutagens and carcinogens (heterocyclic amines, lipid oxides, acrylamides, nitrosamines etc) along with the various metals(cadmium, nickle, aluminum, arsenic, **flouride** etc), plastic toxicities (phthalates etc), pesticides, and herbicidal organophosphates (**glyphosate type chemicals** etc). Then microbes will pass through our bodies without too much of a problem. **Human consciousness to some degree attracts these outbreaks as they are necessary for quicker physical cleansing and evolution** of a degrading species that also exists in a state of biological starvation as it eats cooked food carcinogens daily.

First Pilgrimage (to Italy)

"Heaven and Hell are not physical places but states of mind"

        -Pope John Paul II, 7-28-1999 (paraphrase)

I remember memorizing my first Italian word, "ocho," as I listened to the Italian language tapes that my father had brought home in preparation for our family's Catholic pilgrimage to Rome. I was eight years old and thought it was "neat" that Pope Paul VI and I shared the same name. Even more than the chance to miss a lot of school time, I naturally responded with excitement to a new overseas adventure where I knew things would be different and more interesting. The idea of an overseas trip hit a synchronistic chord in my soul. I was so excited! This would be the first of my many travels and adventures over the next thirty years to Europe, North Africa, and Asia. I later learned that this love of travel or, at least, being more happy away from one's birth area, is common with those who have Uranus rising in their Western geocentric natal birth chart.

During the days before our departure to Italy, I remember worrying inexplicably about the possibility of dying before we left and thus being denied such an exciting adventure. When I shared these feelings with my mother, she very matter-of-factly stated that

I needn't worry about it, as God had other plans for me to fulfill which necessitated my living a longer life. This answer, along with her confident tone of voice, was very satisfying and allowed me to dismiss the death-before-departure scenario. My thoughts clung to her answer again as I experienced the very turbulent Alitalia flight as we slowly flew over the Atlantic Ocean to Rome. Besides, I thought, we were on a Pilgrimage to honor "God" so we would not be permitted to crash. The fact that a Roman Catholic priest was sitting next to me was also reassuring.

The small but memorable things about the trip were the majestic old hotels, churches, cathedrals, fountains, the people on motorbikes, the bitter hot cocoa which needed endless sugar to make it palatable. I was disappointed in the small individual size pizzas which were different than the large American-Italian and Greek-style pizzas back in The States. Of course, the hole-in the-ground ceramic toilets, which I would see in many countries over the years, were also eye-opening.

The pilgrimage involved visiting a few interesting and im-pressive Cathedrals and various outdoor holy sites and a lot of pic-ture taking in the rain with the old style instant Polaroids. These pictures would be scrutinized for vague images formed by darker and lighter patterns which some of the adults called Ahrimanic* or saintly images which gave me an eerie feeling at the time.

Many years later in Asia, I would recall the scrutinization of the Italian holy site pictures as I beheld my first performance of Wayang — the magical shadow puppet plays of Indonesia. As one watches the shadows one soon learns to view them as real charac-ters and forgets that they are just a reflection of the actual marionettes. Even further removed are the strings by which each figure is manipulated and the puppet master himself. What a poignant lesson in life: as a baby grows, the brain inversion subsides, the auric vision fades and the baby is told what to call this or that. Imagination and spiritual connections fade as the parents' realities, worries and thought processes are forced upon infants as though by osmosis — the parents' thought processes become the baby's and their illusions become the baby's realities.

Upon returning from my exotic adventure to my third grade class, I was surprised that everything appeared the same as it had been when I left, even though I was not the same. It was a bit like time travel; I felt that I had changed with this exotic adventure while apparently no one else in my class had. If I had not talked about my trip, no one would know that I had been on, what was to me, such a big adventure. Often I have had similar feelings upon returning to one country from another i.e., that time is indeed relative and it can be used by each in one's own way. Everyone is experiencing one's own karmic path and one may not even care about the experi-ences of others. It is all so personal and appropriate.

*In some Western and Eastern religions and philosophies (including esoteric Christianity), Ahriman is considered to be a post-satanic type energy force which dominates our present evolu-tionary age. Ahrimanic forces promote and thrive on human apathy and materialism (as opposed to satanic energies that thrive on human emotions).

(A beautiful introduction to the study of world philosophies and religion is the greatest philosophical poem of all time: the Indian classic the Bhagavad Gita. The Sankhya system of Kapila, the

4

Yoga philosophy of Patanjali and the Vedas are distinct spiritual streams. In the Bhagavad Gita we have the harmonious presentation of all three spiritual streams. What the Veda philosophy has to give is to be found shining forth in the Bhagavad Gita; what the Yoga of Patanjali has to give mankind we find again in the Bhagavad Gita; and what the Sankhya of Kapila has to give we find there too. The greatness of the Bhagavad Gita lies in the comprehensiveness of its description of how this oriental spiritual life receives its tributaries from the Vedas on the one side, on another from the Sankhya philosophy of Kapila, and again on a third side from the Yoga of Patanjali.)

(*Steiner considers that if man is to rise through Yoga from the ordinary stages of the soul to the higher, he must free himself from external works, he must emancipate himself more and more from outer works, from what he does and perceives externally; he must become a "looker-on" at himself. His soul then assumes an inner freedom and raises itself triumphantly over what is external. That is the case with the ordinary man, but with one who is initiated the case does not remain thus; he is not confronted with external substance, for that in itself is maya. It only becomes a reality to him who makes use of his own inner instruments. Whereas man in everyday life is confronted with substance, with Prakriti—the soul which through Yoga has developed itself by initiation, has to fight against the world of the Asuras, the world of the demoniacal. Substance is what offers resistance; the Asuras become enemies. But all that is as yet a mere suggestion, we perceive it as something we begin to feel which pertains to the soul. For the soul will only begin to realise itself as spiritual when it begins to fight the battle against the demons, the Asuras.

In western thinking Steiner describes this battle as something which becomes perceptible in the form of spirits, when substance appears in spirituality. We thus perceive in miniature that which we know as the battle of the soul-the battle with Ahriman. But when we look upon it as a battle of this kind, we are then in the innermost part of the soul, and what were formerly material spirits grow into something gigantic; the soul is then confronted with the mighty foe. Soul then stands up against Soul, the individual soul in universal space is confronted with the realm of Ahriman. It is the lowest stage of Ahriman's kingdom with which one fights in Yoga; but now when we look at this as the battle of the soul with the powers of Ahriman. Sankhya philosophy recognises this relationship of the soul to external substance, in which the latter has the upper hand, as the condition of Tamas. The initiate who has entered initiation by means of Yoga is not only in this Tamas state, but also in battle with certain demoniacal powers, into which substance transforms itself before his sight. According to Sankhya philosophy, spirit and matter are in balance in the Rajas condition. If this condition is to lead to advancement, it must lead in the sense of the old Yoga to a direct overcoming of Rajas, and lead into Sattva. To us it does not yet lead into Sattva, but to the commencement of another battle-the battle with what is Luciferic.

In Sankhya philosophy Purusha is seen in immense perspective; but if we enter more deeply into that which plays its part in the nature of the soul, not as yet distinguished between Ahriman and Lucifer; then in Sattva, Rajas and Tamas we only find the relation of the soul to material substance. But considering the matter in our own sense, we have the soul in its full activity, fighting and struggling between Ahriman and Lucifer.)

SPAIN

"Siempre hay una sonrisa en el ojo de la mente"
(There is always a smile in the eye of the mind)
This quote reflects the tenacity and hope of the hundreds of Basque political prisoners in jails in 2020- Support the SERA and the *ETXERAT !*

Since my very early years, I have often felt an impatient sense of urgency to go somewhere far away, as though something significant was waiting for me there. I had always treasured my experiences and romanticized my memories. In the 1980s, I finally made the decision again to go abroad. I was bored with college and my life in the States. Most of my friends were foreigners so I figured that overseas I would find more stimulation and more interesting people. After a deliberate five-minute consideration, I decided on Spain as I had some good Latin friends and had always liked the exotic music. I did not go to South America at that time, as it seemed too close to the States geographically, and the fact that it was physically connected to the States only made it less attractive. Therefore, I had rationalized Spain as a Latin alternative and erroneously imagined tanned Latin beauties, passionate people, and good Latin music. I soon learned that Northern Spaniards were light skinned, many blue-eyed and not as emotionally demonstrative as South Americans I had known. Spain's traditional and much of its modern musical style held little attraction for me. Even though much of the local Spanish music was not very inspiring, Spain's legendary gift to humanity

Luis Eduardo Aute's historical concert in Madrid allowed me to hear many Latin international greats like Pablo Milanes, Teddy Bautista, Silvio Rodriguez and Joan Manuel Serrat singing Aute's poignant lyrics and performing music in a truly mesmerizing way that has influenced a 2 generations of anti-Franco Spaniards. Who couldn't be moved listening to Aute's, "De Alguna Manera" or "Al Alba" (dedicated to Franco's last firing squad atrocity).

I ended up in Pamplona, Spain — home of the San Fermines "running of the bulls" festival held during the second week of July each year for one week. This mid-size city swells by tens of thousands as people come from all over the world to participate by "running" with the bulls or just watching the bullfighting, drink the local "Pacharan" (a strong red anise-like drink of Navarre) and eat chorizo sandwiches. Actually, the early morning runs last just a few minutes as the six steers and six bulls run a quick one kilometer into the bullring. This city has prospered much on the yearly summer tourist influx resulting from Hemmingway's portrayal of the Pamplona bullfighting season. There is still a bust of Hemmingway outside of the bullring that, interestingly, is closed for the rest of the year. (The July 2020 running was cancelled.)

I was disillusioned to find the weather in northern Spain, situated in the foothills of the Pyrenees, far from the Mediterranean climate I desired: the cold windy winters without too much snow, the hot humid summers, and the seemingly year-round rain. Finally, after having enough of rainy weekends, a new Japanese friend, who was there on a Mitsubishi-sponsored cultural integration course, and I decided to escape to another country. As France was just a bit north, we headed there. The beautiful bus ride through the western Pyrenees along the Atlantic Ocean was impressive. We were both surprised how pretty and colorful Bayonne and Biaritz in Southwestern France were compared to austere Navarre.

I wondered if I had moved to the wrong country. However, even after hanging out on the topless beaches for a few days and nights and eating our fill of pate on "French" bread, my friend and I had to admit that we preferred the people of Spain as they were nicer and friendlier.

I was fortunate to be in Spain at that time, which was a very energetic, violent, historical few years of significant changes and unknown new freedoms in all aspects of society : sexually (a flood of playboy magazines and public affection was legal), media, schooling, and politics which neither the public or the government could handle. **General Franco had FINALLY died in 1975.** King Juan Carlos was popular and did have a legitimate bloodline claim to the throne and did institute democratic liberal reforms. The first national elections were held in 1981-82. Spain had just entered NATO, and divorce was legalized. Even the Pope (John Paul II) was coming to offer Mass at the Cathedral of Santiago in Galicia, Spain as it was a Catholic year. **Basque language, rights and freedoms had been brutally suppressed by Franco** but had been partially granted in 1980. However, we still lost over 100 brave Basque freedom fighters in 1980. As I was an American, I was particularly valuable in the fight and could travel freely. Sadly, violence and bombings were still being carried out by ETA, the Basque freedom fighters/separatist group.

Police still carried machine guns and interesting anti-American war eagle posters were seen alongside the Basque independence slogans written in the linguistically unique Euskara language. Having been a supporter of Irish Freedom fighters against the British for so many years, supporting the Basque movement and Batsuna was somehow familiar. Whether it is supporting the Irish, Basques, or human rights in S.E. Asia in the 1990s, a young innocent looking-American with a valid passport can be of huge assistance.

My Second Pilgrimage — Santiago, Spain

St. James (Santiago), the suppossed apostle of "Jesus of Nazareth", is the Patron Saint of Spain. His remains are said to lay in the Catedral de Santiago de Compostela in Galicia, Spain. As 1982 was a Catholic holy year (a year when St. James' Day falls on a Sunday), Pope John Paul II (who was also, interestingly, from a state in Poland called Galicia) was coming to Santiago to celebrate Mass in the local dialect called Gallego. In years past, hundreds of thousands are said to have taken the sacred pilgrimage to the Cathedral of Santiago (often starting from Paris) in either sincere religious fervor or as part of their criminal sentence during the Middle Ages.

Our rainy pilgrimage was done by car, bike, and foot. I did not actually qualify for the Compostela (certificate) from the Cathedral. In order to receive a Compostela, one must walk at least 100km (60 miles) or bike 200km in one stretch. Few Americans reach this special out-of-the-way pilgrimage spot in Galicia in Northwestern Spain. After 1986, the number of Spaniards walking on the pilgrimage began to increase dramatically. In 1999, the Last Holy Year, 150,000 "Compostelas" were recorded by the Cathedral Society— mostly to Spaniards followed by French and other Europeans.

To me the debate among academics as to whether St James's existed or his body actually made it to Santiago is not as important as the consideration that anytime thousands of people concentrate their energy in any one place over many years, it clearly allows for an energy vortex to develop as in Santiago. One could feel this energy in the air in Santiago — I felt it as peaceful and heavy at the same time as though it was forcing me to slow down and reflect on history. It was a perfect atmospheric setting to be exposed to such strong spiritual energies.

I was lucky to have been able to attend, through some Opus Dei* friends, Pope John Paul II's Mass in the legendary Cathedral of Santiago. The King and Queen of Spain were also in attendance. This pilgrimage, the setting of narrow brick-lined streets, misty weather, the long conversations in the local bars while munching on lots of peppered cut pieces of octopus and the history-imbued area are all still peacefully refreshing to recall. I would return to do another pilgrimage to Santiago a few years later in an attempt to deal with some personal issues. This poignant experience would allow me years later to readily understand the need for my father's pilgrimage to Jerusalem as part of his spiritual preparation for his death.

It was while I was living in Spain that I first made friends with some Japanese people who impressed me and aroused my curiosity even more about their culture. It is interesting in hindsight to note that many years later when I did move to Japan, the first Japanese Doctor of Acupuncture that allowed me to work with him in Japan as a professional equal was a man who had been living in Mallorca, Spain in 1982 when I had been there. This allowed us to communicate in Spanish before my Japanese improved. This doctor epitomized what would become my positive image of Japanese who go abroad and develop resilience and mental flexibility (hard to acquire inside such a homogenous country like Japan ruled by such a patronizing bureaucracy) while retaining all the more subtle beautiful human qualities that I would discover in so many Japanese people.

*(Opus Dei is a very unique organization as it is the only "personal prelature" in the Roman Catholic Church i.e., a world dioceses whose head (prelate) reports directly to the Pope. Its founder, Saint José Marie Escriva de Balaguer was canonized in 2002 (which was only 27 years after he died and is the fastest canonization in history). All the people I have met associated with their work were sincere and very dedicated individuals. An Opus Dei priest is rumored to be a candidate for the next Pope.)

The goal of freeing 460 of the Basque political prisoners still in 73 jails in France and Spain continues even now in 2020. Please support the SERA and the ETXERA ! Google "ARGIA"

Japan Bound

"Audentis fortuna iuvat "(fortune favors the bold)
                                                    -Virgil

As I prepared to board the plane for the sixteen-hour flight from the States to Tokyo, I knew instinctively that I was heading in the right direction. Although initially I had considered other Asian countries, my difficulty with the Sino-Tibetan tonal languages like Chinese and Thai had made my decision to go to Japan that much easier (for most people I know, Japanese, an Altaic language, is much easier to learn). Japan was also convenient because even though I was prepared to study any style of martial art provided the teacher was exceptional, the style I had been training in the States was considered to be a "Japanese" style.

I had US$2,000 and some yen in my pocket and no credit cards. I felt that this journey was part of my karmic unfoldment. I had finished my graduate training and internship in Oriental medicine, achieved my childhood goal of "shodan" (martial artist 1st degree black belt) degree and had studied various Oriental subjects in both undergraduate and graduate schools in the States and Europe. Yet, I was still insecure and knew that I needed to keep looking elsewhere for something that would make me feel more complete and happy. Local USA acupuncture clinics were inadequate to offer a large patient load and hospitals were not contracting acupuncturists.

I still had no idea where to stay once I got through customs and took the two-hour bus ride into Tokyo. I had become accustomed in most western international cities to just using the airport city guides and pension services to find a place to stay (usually downtown) and thus little planning was necessary. This informal style works well as it allows one to mix with other foreigners and exchange information at places frequented by experienced travelers who are usually very savvy about local updated pertinent information. However, in Tokyo this did not work so well, since there are 30 million people in greater Tokyo and many areas that foreigners would call downtown areas. Most of the airport information pertains to luxury hotels or boring sterile business hotels where I knew I could never mix and get useful information. Many of these hotels are located in the less attractive business areas (such as Shinagawa) which have little of interest to most newcomers.

As the pilot announced that we would soon be landing at Tokyo's Narita Airport, I suddenly felt a surge of panic about not having any place to stay so I pulled out my outdated guidebook and decided to head for the Shinjuku area in northwestern central Tokyo. The Shinjuku area proved to be a good call. It is located in the more modern western half of Tokyo, which most foreigners prefer and conveniently located on many subway lines and at least 12 above ground train lines. I have often thought how lucky I was to have not chosen one of the many bleak unexciting areas inside Tokyo such as Shinagawa that would have been very discouraging.

It was a hot August Saturday evening and as I got off the 2,300-yen, two-hour bus ride from the airport, I was a bit overwhelmed by the huge crowds, traffic, humidity and multi-story buildings with illegible neon signs in "kanji" "hiragana" and "katakana." "Kanji" are what most call the pictographic Chinese writing. "Hiragana" and "katakana" are simple alphabetic-type abbreviated scripts that are also of Chinese kanji origin but can be memorized in one day. The Japanese took just a few thousand of the kanji from the Chinese system and added katakana for grammatical endings and kanji clarification. "Katakana" was also known as "kanbun" or Chinese Literature as this script was used by the Japanese aristocracy to study the Chinese Classical texts. "Hiragana" was traditionally known as "wabun," meaning Japanese literature or "onnade," meaning woman's hand as it was used mainly by woman (who wrote some of the most important Japanese literature) and did not require the use of "kanji."

A Japanese student needs to learn only 1800 kanji to graduate from high school and 3200 kanji for college. However, Japanese grammar is very complex. The Chinese language is grammatically simple but has thousands more kanji and a complex intonation/tone system that I found difficult.

I was determined to stay somewhere local and interesting as opposed to a regular expensive hotel as I knew that there were many "gaijin" (foreigner) houses that rented more traditional rooms. I had not come to Tokyo, as so many Westerners, to do some boring materialistic business job such as finance or computers that I saw at that time in my life as contributing little to human consciousness. No! I had come to accelerate my karmic path which, judging from my life choices and interests, was intimately tied to Asia. I assumed that it would be an easy society for me to adapt to as I had been "training" for it at different levels consciously and unconsciously for years.

I finally figured out how to use the public phone and called a few outdated numbers until I found a place to stay. Optimistically content that I had communicated a bit on the phone, i.e. I could ask questions in Japanese but not understand the answer (a common problem for me), I went to grab the first cab I saw and suddenly realized that I had cut to the front of the longest cab line I had ever seen in my life. However, the people in the front of the line practically pushed me into the cab obviously having sympathy for an overdressed, sweating tourist with luggage who obviously did not know what was going on. I thought how nice they were and how patiently they all waited; I would get much needed practice in the development of the virtue of patience in Japan.

Soon I was in my first hostel-like abode called a "gaijin house" in a very lively part of Tokyo known as "shin-okubo." After the motherly manager scolded me for wasting money on a cab when the "hostel" was one train stop from where I had just called, I was shown to a very, very small private room (maybe three meters by two meters). There was a small hole-in-the-ground ceramic common toilet and shower in the hallway (always separate, of course, as it is considered unrefined to have a bath for cleansing and a toilet for defecation in the same room). I soon met another American staying there and learned from him that the job ads would, conveniently, be out the next day in Monday's largest English newspaper, the "Japan Times." This American was interesting as he was really "into" everything Japanese. I would meet others like him over the years who tried to mimic all the little learned mannerisms, taught nuances and intonations (which Japanese people usually use in public) which seemed silly and unnatural to me for a Japanese let alone a Westerner. It seemed that they really wanted to be as Japanese-like as possible and awkwardly did not fit into the Western environment in which they had been raised.

They did not socialize well with Westerners in Japan. Other such people dealing with similar identity issues seemed to be rejecting aspects of Western life that they saw as wrong or inferior by becoming as "unwestern" as possible.

There were places everywhere with delicious food— an epicurean's delight! Fortunately, for newcomers and kanji illiterates like myself, there were plastic models of some of the offered dishes outside most restaurants enabling one to drag the waitress outside and point to what one wanted to eat. I quickly learned the food essentials such as "cha-han" (fried rice), "ramen" (spaghetti-type noodle soup), katsu-don" (fried pork on a bed of rice) etc.... Most of the everyday, informal places to eat at were more Chinese-style rice/noodle dishes with the real Japanese-style places being more expensive and not as fast (except for the inexpensive rotating sushi bars).

I knew that I would have to act quickly to find work before my three-month tourist visa expired and I ran out of money. My US$2,000 would not last long as just a very small one room (six tatami-mat size) apartment went for around US$800 a month.

I was lucky in that before 1990 a foreigner could, after finding an employer willing to sponsor him by guaranteeing him a monthly salary of 250,000 yen (US$2000), get the work-visa stamp placed in his passport right in Tokyo. After 1990* there was another seemingly anti-foreigner rule instituted which necessitated that all foreigners travel to a Japanese embassy or consulate outside of Japan to get their work-visa. This meant that after going to the expense and usual hassles of relocating to Japan and finding work independently, you would have to take another overseas trip to the Japanese embassy in Seoul or Hong Kong (South Korea was the closest and most inexpensive at around US$200-300 roundtrip) to receive the one year work-visa stamp in your passport and then return to Tokyo. This rule change was odd by modern international standards and was interpreted by foreigners as an attempt to limit the influx of what the Japanese government saw as too many undesirable foreigners. (In reality, even as late as 2003, foreigners constituted a whopping 1.4% of the total Japanese population and two-thirds of this 1.4% were Chinese.(1) Still, Japan had become the "new frontier" for immigrants seeking fortunes both legally and illegally which provided a very interesting atmosphere for foreigners, like myself, to interact and learn from each other. In January of 2004, the national NHK news station aired that the Japanese government announced a plan to reduce illegal immigration by 50% by 2005.) This rule change seemed to be directed at the Southeast Asian influx who worked the booming construction trade as well as the large increase in Iranians who often sold illegal drugs and prepaid illegal phone cards. These illegal phone cards were sold at a 90% discount and used by

(The immigration rules were changed in 2003 so one no longer has to leave the country to get a work-visa. A new large immigration building opened in Shinagawa in 2003 to serve foreigners living in the greater Tokyo area; inconveniently, three other local offices were closed.) many foreigners for overseas calls on the many international public phones all over the big cities. This was big business. The use of these "illegal" phone cards became so prevalent due to the very expensive monopolized KDD international phone rates that by 1995 most of the many public international phones were adjusted so that they could not take any phone cards; a major inconvenience to many. Fortunately, new less expensive international phone carriers started to appear so one could say that the

Iranians unwittingly instituted an opening of the communication markets for all foreigners.

This repeated pattern of forced changes, initiated by foreigners unwilling to subject themselves to what they perceived as an unfair or overpriced social/business environment in Japan, resulted in many positive changes for the Japanese people. It also forced Japan to internationalize more and be less patronizing toward its citizens.

However, for most foreigners new visa stipulations were just a minor inconvenience. Westerners easily forged university degrees (only copies were usually necessary) required to get work-visas. The Israelis controlled most of the very lucrative street selling of jewelry and made plenty of money to show customs proof of fi-nancial resources needed to repeatedly come and go every three months on tourist-visas. This "street selling" was a very profitable business and the prime selling areas near certain train stations such as Shinjuku or Ueno were rented for thousands of dollars monthly by Israelis from other Israelis who paid off the "Yakuza" (Japanese organized crime groups).

Thai and Mexican silver jewelry was very popular among Japanese as they are a people who resonate with lunar-type vibrations such as rice (the national staple), the cherry blossom tree (the national tree) and silver; all three are main moon correspondences in certain astrological systems. This astrological connection is an interesting explanation as to why the Japanese kept paying incredibly inflated prices for nice but actually very low wholesale cost silver in the 1990s.

Street selling was very professionally handled and everyone was profiting except the Japanese consumer who paid exorbitant prices. Most Israelis had no real interest or means to get a sponsored work-visa as that meant a boring company job. Israelis usually came over after doing their mandatory national army service, worked the street stalls, saved a lot of money, vacationed in S.E. Asia and eventually returned home. This was a gold mine for many hard working Israelis willing to work the streets. Two of my close Israeli friends each saved over US$100,000 in just 2-3 years.

What really stood-out about the Israelis I met all over Asia was how attractive they were. The intermarriage between so many different peoples had obviously produced quick-thinking, physically nice-looking people. It would have been easy for me to have gotten caught-up in their nomadic comfortable gypsy-type life style. Had I not been so serious about my training schedule in Japan at that time, I would have easily been enticed by my Israeli girlfriend to follow her to a new life in Southern India. However, as my life in East Asia was just beginning, I decided to stay in Japan. I also felt at that time that if I went to India with her, I would be entering a very different karmic path that would have been a long term distraction, albeit a pleasant one, from what I saw as my immediate life task.

The Southeast Asian workers in Japan were not as lucky as they worked long hard paid hours albeit underpaid by Japanese standards. The men often did city construction or countryside factory work and the women often did various types of hostess work. Many a third-world family was supported and houses bought by yen remittances from hard-working, self-sacrificing foreigners. According to the Philippine Overseas Employment Administration, Philippinos' total overseas remittances averaged US$8 billion during the 1990's and the largest percentage of this came from those working in Japan — representing the major source of revenue for the Philippines. It was the only country in Southeast Asia with no economic growth and only 10-20% of other S.E. Asian tourist inflow. (2) I remember a really sweet Philippina friend stoically telling me how sad she was that her brothers back home in Cebu were using her hard-earned hostess income to drink and gamble and that no one in her large family was working since she started sending money home. She herself lived with many other Philippinas in a tiny old shabby apartment provided by their employer. She refused all my urging to save money for herself and stop remittances for a while. There were so many similar cases that, albeit exasperating, admiringly reflected a level of sacrifice and humility that demanded respect and which most developed countries' people could not bear.

The Japanese government, in an apparent attempt to limit unruly foreigners but still fill the need for cheap labor, decided in 1990 to give all South Americans with proven Japanese ancestry a two year work-visa as opposed to the standard one-year visa. I assumed that the government correctly figured that those of Japanese descent would be a more homogenous and controllable lot. All jobs and visas were planned in Brazil and Peru. Sao Paolo, Brazil has over one million Brazilians of Japanese descent (most had migrated from Japan in the late 19th and early 20th century and restructured and built-up Brazil's agricultural scene). **In just a few years, 150,000 Brazilians and 30,000 Peruvians flooded into Japan in just a few years. (3)**

The South Americans with college educations were placed in city professional jobs, and the less educated were placed in rural factories. I had Latin friends doing both computer jobs in the city and factory jobs out in the country. The Brazilians proved to be a positive influence as they ran many fun nightclubs and restaurants and had little of the violent illegal tendencies shown by some of the Iranians and the Chinese triads. I spent many a pleasant night in these fun salsa clubs that also provided a memorable place to experience the World Cup and soccer frenzy that spread across Japan in the early 1990's.

I was on the train in Tokyo on March 20th 1995 when five two-man terrorist teams from the Aum Shinrikyo religious cult, riding on separate subway trains, converged at the Kasumigaseki station and secretly release lethal sarin gas into the air. The terrorists then took a sarin antidote and escaped while the commuters, blinded and gasping for air, rushed to the exits. Twelve people died, and 5,500 were treated in hospitals, some in a comatose state. Most of the survivors recovered, but some victims suffered permanent damage to their eyes, lungs, and digestive systems. If the sarin gas had been disseminated more effectively at Kasumigaseki station, a hub of the Tokyo subway system, tens of thousands might have been killed. The Japanese police raided Aum Shinrikyo headquarters and arrested hundreds of members, including the cult's blind leader, Shoko Asahara.

For most Japanese people, the violent world was a separate world typical of foreigners. Generally, my impression was that Japanese felt safe and protected inside Japan and out-of-place and vulnerable outside Japan. I remember how impressed I was the first time I saw a Japanese sleeping late at night on a train (sober or not) obviously not concerned about being robbed. This is but one of many examples which over the years caused me to feel an increased sense of security and increased sense of relaxation in Japan. Although I enjoyed this relaxation to a degree, I also associated it, long-term, with a decreased sense-of-alertness, quickness of thinking and an undermining of an aspect of mental acuity necessary in life outside of Japan. Fortunately, my personal training and travels allowed me to keep my survival mentality alive and well in a healthful way. Overall, I saw very little overt violence in Japan. I would occasionally encounter some of the boisterous right-wing extremists or vapid yakuza street boys. I soon learned it was useless to try to reason with them. At such times, I had no choice but to act in a non-passive way.

One of many incidents that stand out for its blatant xenophobic sentiment was the time a drunken Japanese guy tried to stab me with a hunting knife on a train to Omiya. I was sitting on an uncrowded night train with no one on either side of me and this odd-looking guy sitting across from me and talking to himself stood up and came to sit right next to me. I slid down away from him. He slowly took out a hunting knife, showed it to me and asked me if I liked it. I just stared at him and said, "urusai yo," indicating that he was bothering me. The next thing I knew he was lunging at me with the knife. Fortunately, I was able to disarm him, but the police were waiting at the next train stop and as I was a foreigner holding a knife, they initially reacted against me until I angrily explained, with the support of some of the other locals who saw the whole incident. It turned out that this assailant just did not like foreigners. However, as so often happened in Japan, because the assailant was drunk and I was not really hurt (I only needed a few stitches), the police negotiated a payment to be made by him to me — end of case — no prosecution. I agreed to meet him in a coffee house of my choosing (what a concession!) to finalize the settlement. Actu-ally, this was all quite interesting and odd as I thought about meet-ing one's assailant for coffee. However, I greedily recalled reading about similar payments of large sums of money being paid to an offended party. I cheerfully decided to ask for five million yen (US $50,000). As it turned out, the guy was unemployed, basically broke, and his wife refused to help him out much so we settled on US$5,000. He was very apologetic, meek and bowed his head a lot (a good strategy for "disarming" the other person, as I almost felt bad for this seemingly servile man). Many jail sentences are avoided in Japan if the crime is committed under the influence of alcohol, and an apology is expressed. **An apology is very significant in Japan and one often sees public apologies with much bowing on T.V. news** shows. Even though most foreigners dismiss this apologetic ritual as insincere and superficial, a pertinent recent case of murder, in August of 2003, enforces the reality that for some Japanese an apol-ogy has deep meaning. The case involved the murder of a journalist and author, Satoru Someya, who wrote about Tokyo's (Shinjuku's) Kabuki-cho criminal underworld. A Japanese man who, according to a Kyodo News story on 1-16-2004, had been offended by things Someya San wrote about him in a just published book and recent magazine article, kidnapped Someya-San and after he refused to apologize for things he had written, brutally stabbed him to death and dumped his body in Tokyo Bay. I, like many others, wrongly assumed that it had been a Chinese organized killing. The point due consideration is that not only did the murderer demand an apology but that the author refused to give him something so seemingly simple which possibly could have spared his life.

The uninvestigated murders of some overseas hostesses and call-girls were not reported much in the Japanese press but were widely known and discussed among most Southeast Asian people whom I knew. Missing friends and abusive employers were com-mon topics at a counseling centre for foreigners where I had the emotional experience of working in the early 1990's. Many of those missing, as well as their friends, had illegally overstayed their entertainment-visas (commonly used by Southeast Asians to gain ac-cess to Japan) in Japan and felt they had no practical legal recourse. I can poignantly recall a close friend tearfully writing a letter to the family of her friend who had been missing for one month and was assumed dead. The family sent a letter back to my friend stoically thanking her for her kindness stating they knew things could end up in such a way.

The government always presented AIDS as a reason to be wary of foreigners and as further evidence of dirty foreigners versus hygienic Japanese (this has some historic validity, as the Japanese have always been a particularly hygienic people, and this is very noticeable when traveling around much of Asia nowadays or apparently even 100 years ago as numerous historical accounts attest to. Mainland China, especially, is where newcomers often find it hard to stand what is considered unrefined or crude in more developed countries e.g, the common practice in many places of openly spitting sea-food shells or anything else on the floor while eating so that one cannot walk around the table without practically slipping). The birth-control pill was finally "approved" or legalized officially in Japan in 2000 but is neither in demand (only an estimated 1%) or encouraged as it could probably lead to an increased rate of sexually transmitted disease.

The whole sophomoric sex-for-money scene in Japan seemed to have a child-like non-passionate almost innocent quality to it. Foreigners are often surprised by the large number of "soap houses," live audience participating sex shows (no foreigner participation allowed) and persistent daily mail-ads they receive for call-girl services in Tokyo. (Still, this was not as blatant as the direct phone calls I got daily in Chinese hotels from call-girls which, I suppose, one can use a chance to practice the local dialect.

One sex tour in China in September 2003 received media attention in Asia (including Japan) and alerted many to how large a problem this is as it involved 400 Japanese male employees and 500 Chinese prostitutes. The fact that the 3-day "tour" ended on the anniversary of the Japanese invasion of N.E. China (on 9-18-1931) was seen as a calculated insult by the both the Chinese government and many people. The 5-star hotel in Zhuhai, Guangdong Province in southeastern China was closed for months while the Chinese police investigated. An article in the Mainichi newspaper reported, in January 2004, that the Chinese courts sentenced 14 Chinese nationals to jail time, including two people for life, for organizing the event.

When I was working in a clinic in "Kabuki-cho" (an area of Shinjuku with a lot of adult clubs) about 10% (a large statistical percentage) of the foreign girls in the huge sex industry we saw tested positive for HIV. Most of these were very young child-like girls recruited from Southeast Asia (Philippines and Thailand) and some harder-edged girls from Colombia. A 2001 Japanese government white paper reported that of the 1,516 HIV-infected women infected in Japan in 2002, 1,090 were foreigners; of women with full-blown AIDS, two-thirds were foreign. Japan's Health and Welfare Ministry 2003 figures put the number of HIV and AIDS cases together at only 8000. Compared to almost a million estimated cases for North America and 550,000 for Western Europe, this number is still small but does show a 23% increase since 2001-2002. With its $13 billion a year sex industry growing (7), a 25% drop in condom use in the 1990's (according to Japan's largest condom manufacturers), newly legalized birth control pills, and low government education intervention, the World Health Organization has cited Japan as a country of great concern.(8)

It is interesting to note that by 2018 the Japanese government's top concerns are Japan's rapid population decline (1.4 births per woman well below the base replacement rate of 2.1) and a 20 year ongoing recession. Even though there is a worldwide population decline concern by 2018, Japan's 2050 population projection of 100 million , down from 130 million in 2017 is alarming and is a crisis. In 2016, Japan's Diet (congress) decided to quickly enact new legislation to allow immigrants to more easily come to and work and stay in Japan. Also removing the Japanese language proficiency test that was prohibitive for many . This is a huge change. Most of these newer visas are for SE Asians in limited skill jobs. The goal was to attract 345,000 new foreign workers and it was largely successful by 2020.

REFERENCES

1. Japanese Government Handbook of Statistics. 2003 Kudansha Tokyo,
   Japan

2. French Agency Presse, 8-26-2001 issue.

3. Japanese Government Handbook of Statistics. 2002 Kudansha Tokyo,
   Japan

4. "Hong Kong Triad and Japanese Yakuza Forming Crime Alliance,"
   Deutsche Presse-   Agentur, December 13, 1999

5. Asiaweek, May 9, 1997 issue (national section) pg 63

6. Robin Morgan, Sisterhood Is Global (New York: Feminist Press of the
   City University of New York, 1996)

6. Coalition Against Trafficking in Women-Asia Pacific, "Prostitution in
   Asia," August 8, 1999

7. Velisarios, Kattoulas, "Slaves of Tokyo," Times (London), January 27,
   2001

8. "W.H.O. Notes Lucrative Asian Sex Trade," Business World, August 31,
   2001

INITIATION

Soon after arriving in Tokyo, I began making the rounds of different Japanese clinics without any formal invitation. I was surprised at how nice everyone was despite their initial confusion at my inadequate Japanese and the novelty of a foreign acupuncturist. I continued this informal style of work for months as I was often invited to observe, help and even apprentice but not actually work as a professional equal. I decided it best to just apprentice for a while and learn the local scene. Being an apprentice at many places meant doing various acu-points on patients until the organ arterial pulses changed before progressing to more refined treatments. As Japanese acupuncture schools do not teach herbology, the acupuncture training and techniques are much more comprehensive than in Chinese schools where herbology is emphasized over needling techniques. There are many effective Japanese "modern" (post WWII) acupuncture techniques not widely taught in the States. However, more schools in the States are now offering Japanese courses than when I went to school in the 1980s.

I found some Japanese techniques intellectually challenging and theoretically beautiful. Clinically, these techniques are very effective done properly, as they move an aspect of energy in unique ways that would not normally occur in the body's standard meridian system. **This energy is known as "ki" in Japan, "chi" in China and "prana" in India.** The Chinese and Japanese use the same kanji/character for "ki" or "chi" as in their word for electricity that is pronounced "<u>de</u>**ki**" in Japanese. These different, and in my opinion, stronger acupuncture techniques also demand a greater degree of responsibility of the clinician. I am sure that more schools will soon be teaching these Japanese techniques as part of their curriculum instead of just a one-time seminar. Many patients respond better to one style than another so it only makes sense that one learns Japanese as well as other styles of acupuncture.

One hot humid summer evening, as I was walking to the train station in Tokyo after another day of routine clinical work, I decided to take a different way to the station hoping to find a new place to try for dinner. With dozens of restaurants near all major stations, this was an easy and fun thing to do. Since it was so hot, I wanted some fresh fire-cooked eel (a popular summer dish as it has a cooling effect on the body). I soon found myself lost a bit (another easy thing to do) and in view of a temple that I had not seen before. In Japanese, the word "Otera" implies a Buddhist temple as opposed to the word "Jinzya" which implies a Shinto shrine; these two terms often confuse foreigners. Since I usually stopped in a new temple when I found one, I decided to let the eel wait and to make a visit. This practice became almost a daily ritual, as it felt especially good, as my meditations done on temple grounds were so vivid. The interesting thing was that I was the only layperson ever there. The monks who unusually wore various color robes and hairstyles, just acted as though I was not there except for the usual little nod now and then that let me know that I was welcome.

After many months of visiting this particular temple, a monk came over and asked if he could sit with me. It was my birthday. This monk invited me to have some tea with him and his seniors. I knew this was considered to be a special meeting as we sat drinking "gyo-kuro" tea (the top of the line "uji-cha" tea) on a table made of a beautiful wood I had not seen before but I would later identify in China as zitan (a type of wood highly prized in Asia). My new monk friend, who told me to call him simply (and informally) Amsa, informed me that he was a lay Buddhist and had trained in China with a Charn sect* and that others in his group were from a Mikkyou sect* and a Kagyu Sect*. Hearing this clarified the variation in robe types, colors and hair length that I had been wondering about; usually one group wore the same color robes and hairstyle. Amsa explained that his group had trained in what I would know as various metaphysical and martial arts but the monks just called all such studies "laws of nature." Amsa said that the monks had been watching me after they also noticed that no one else ever came onto the temple grounds when I was there. He told me that one of the monks had had a confirmatory dream that indicated that I was in their karmic group from past lives in Mongolia. I accepted this as an interesting possibility, as I had had many disturbing dreams over the years that I had always figured were residual hangover memories from disturbances encountered in some violent Asian setting in a past life. The karmic group theory was a possible explanation for my attraction to and perseverance in the martial arts and Asian studies. It also would help explain why mare's milk was, while odd-tasting for sure, somehow thirst quenching to me while others on my first trip to China in 1989 would spit it out in disgust (Mare's milk was a dietary staple for many warring Mongols and others in the plains and conferred to them greatly needed strength).

The "Elders" (again we had no honorific terms to denote one's standing but various acknowledged status was obvious) would later explain that residual emotions from my violent nomadic past lives were so deeply engrained on my nervous system during those past lives that they were still housed in my subtle bodies* in this incarnation. In metaphysical thought, most past life hangover energies should be cleared-out so that one can free oneself from various karmic strands. **All frictional karmic threads properly released allow one to receive higher refined energies more easily which will strengthen the physical body and prepare one, eventually, to receive the even higher spiritual energies.** These higher energies tend to deplete and weaken the average physical body due to its high degree of toxicity and impaired nervous system resulting from modern cooked food diets. The Elders would facilitate this energetic attunement for me along with much else over the next many years.

This memorable birthday began many years of enhanced training into esoteric aspects of healing and energetics that would lead me to other Asian countries in search of additional clarification and understanding. It was all I had hoped for and more— to be able to travel within Asia while training in martial arts and doing various healing work in so many clinics.

The poverty, abuses, post-war and drug-related sadness that exists in Southeast Asia is mind-numbing. Seeing such tragedy and sadness has really kept things in perspective as I have gone through life. More poignant still, are the ready smiles and expressive love on children's faces, despite such suffering and lack of expectations.

I loved the food in the various Asian countries to which I went. The people, overall, were very nice, even sweet and sincere — unspoiled by Western standards. Sadly, it soon became appar-ent that, generally, the Japanese were the least happy, and most prosperous, of all Asian people that I met. There were so many instances outside of Japan, even amidst poverty and disease, where spontaneous looks on people's faces, gestures, and words reflected happiness and a sincere desire to help. Instances like this were all too rare in Japan.

I was not surprised to read, in a 2002 Japanese newspaper, that the Japanese Ministry of Health, Welfare and Labour determined that the suicide rate had increased to 31,042 in 2001—which was 85 suicides a day, twice the per capita suicide rate in the States. Of course, with the mental health field/ professions being so undeveloped in Japan, getting help for the depressed or traumatized is difficult. There are now some antidepressants and antipsychotics on the Japanese market.

Charn (Zen in Japan) is considered the first Chinese Buddhist sect (as opposed to Indian). The original Indian style of Buddhism was adapted to better suit the Chinese people. The Charn sect was not as conservative as many of the other sects and, thus, attracted a wide variety of people such as warrior/monks and various artists who other sects would not permit to enter.

Shingon or colloquially "Mikkyou" is an eclectic Japanese Buddhist order based on Tibetan Buddhism. Many energy healers, like the recently popular but poorly and quickly trained Reiki practitioners in the States, borrow from some of these Indian based teachings.

Kagyu is one the four traditional Tibetan Buddhist Orders whose high Lama (analogous to the Catholic Pope) is known as the Karmapa (there has been much controversy and intrigue over the present 17th Karmapa as there are two adherents to the title and the Dalai Lama unusually weighed in and showed a preference for one candidate over the other; this is like non-Catho-lic Christians choosing the Catholic Pope). The well-known Dalai Lama is the high lama of the Gelug order which stresses academic Buddhist scripture study. The Kagyu sects tend to emphasize meditation and other more esoteric aspects of Buddhism. The other two traditional sects are called Sakya and Nyingma. All Tibetan Buddhist orders have had headquarters in Northern India since the in-famous massacre of Tibetans by the Chinese in 1959. (The Chinese takeover of Tibet began officially in 1950.)

  *In metaphysical literature the human body is usually divided into 7-12 subtle "layers" of a more etheric nature which lie outside of our physical body. These **subtle bodies** relate to how we receive energy from the higher aspects of our soul and spirit. Refer to Dr. Rudolph Steiner's Anthroposophical Approach to Medicine Anthroposophical Press. 1957

  ***Chakras** are considered to be energy vortices in our subtle bodies that connect with the physical body and adjust higher vibra-tional energies. There are seven main chakras that relate to our seven main endocrine glands and their related organs. Overall, there are 360 chakras as seen to be the main acupuncture points. See Alice Bailey, Esoteric Healing N.Y. Lucis Publishing Co., 1980.

Martial Art Training

As I had done, most older boys in the U.S.A. initially enroll in martial art training of their own volition for the simple reason of being able to defend themselves; which at its core is a motivation based on fear. As one progresses with proper training, the many benefits of increased confidence can be enjoyed, and this is beautiful to both feel in oneself as well as behold in others, especially one's students or children. It is interesting to note that much of this newfound confidence is usually, in actuality, not reality based i.e., the student may not really be able to defend themselves physically in many situations (as many, like myself, learn in their first real fight after starting training). However, they have become more familiar with fighting techniques, being hit, and striking others in a controlled fun environment on a regular basis and so the idea of a fight is not as closely associated in their thinking with the unknown or fear. Of course, there has been some increase in skill, strength, coordination and, thus, fighting ability but, the main change has been in one's thinking. After many years, some will actually be able to fight well, but almost everyone will certainly be able to fight better or at least defend oneself in a more skilled manner than when they started training. For me, the actual fear of being hit and hurt has always been both a motive for more training as well as a fear that I erroneously thought would go away after many years of training. Despite having trained many of my body parts to withstand direct punches and kicks, this fear persisted. It was merely the fear-based anticipation before the altercation started and was gone once the challenge commenced. This has taught me much about the illusion of fear. In Japan, this self-defense/fear motive is not the main reason for initial training as physical fights are much less common in school.

Most Japanese also start martial art training for increased confidence that an improved mind and body will confer, but without actually anticipating the need for fighting in the streets. This fear factor is a major difference between the initial motivations of most people in the States and in Japan to start martial art training. Of course, as one continues to train, or for those who were originally of a more refined nature, one learns to appreciate both the more subtle attributes which flower through many years of training as well as the direct connection to nature, earth and its implosive energy potential which can be tapped into through the martial arts.

I was a 1st degree black belt ("shodan") in a Chinese/Okinawa karate style when I arrived in Japan. Despite what many think, a black belt does not confer expertise. It takes three to five years in many traditional karate systems to qualify for a 1st degree black belt and then another three to five years for a 2nd degree ("nidan") and then roughly five years for each further advancement. Most Chinese styles do not use belts as rankings, but most Japanese styles do use them. One of the martial art centers ("dojo" in Japanese but this word is often understood in many countries) in Asia at which I did physical training was in a Buddhist temple in Japan. As I had trained in this style for many years, the elders thought it wise to continue with the same style for further physical strengthening. I am honored to be associated with the Uehara family who are well respected in Japan. I would continue to train under

Master Uehara in Tokyo for ten years when I was not working or training in China, Malaysia, Singapore, Thailand, or Hong-Kong. Martial training at this dojo required a lot of physical strength that built up the energy or "chi" in the arms, legs and stomach first and later in more sensitive areas such as the neck, ribs and groin. It is always such a joy and privilege to be a part of a group that allows for both one's own healthfully selfish concentration of energy for one's personal growth and goals as well as shared group energy that all can utilize. This energy becomes stronger if the same actions are repeated many times in the same place. Such training creates a type of energy vector that can accelerate one's progress even more if one consciously taps into it. People naturally do this to various extents unconsciously in non-training areas of life.

Most of the martial art dojo where I trained were such a place of group energy sharing. Very little selfish ego came into play as everyone eagerly helped everyone else knowing that each was at one's own level of power and skill and just trying to get better at one aspect or another over time. The power that I have seen at various dojo in Asia could make many a man arrogant and aggressive were he not properly trained.

The martial art training in China usually starts much younger than in Japan and produces very versatile well-rounded martial artists who know many styles and weapons. Most Chinese martial artists I know are generally physically more coordinated, graceful and flexible than Japanese martial artists. This is readily apparent to anyone who observes a stereotypical hard, tight Japanese karate form compared to a stereotypical rhythmical, more acrobatic type Chinese kung-fu form.

It is interesting to contrast the graceful methodical movements of an "internal" Chinese martial art such as "Tai chi chuan" to the apparent crudeness of a Thai style kickboxing match. In Bangkok, one can watch many kickboxing competitions, as there are Thai kickboxing fights almost nightly at one of two different stadiums. Most foreigners are surprised how young the teenage competitors are at most of these fights and how bloody they can become. Many of these young fighters are not particularly strong or technically orientated, but the rawness and endurance seen is inspiring and real. Eventually some become excellent mature fighters (My bruised body found out the hard way in Bangkok that I needed a lot more training).

Many martial artists believe that both extremes need to be developed to really master any martial art. It is interesting to note that most people initially study one of the so-called "harder external" styles of karate (Uechi-ryu) or kung-fu (crane) to increase youthful confidence and fighting skills. Eventually, however, many turn to the Chinese internal styles such as **"Tai chi chuan"** **"Ba-kua" or "Hsing-yi"** to learn what they did not learn from the external styles or enhance what they did learn. From a health perspective it is indeed wise to study the internal forms as such training with the emphasis on breathing, rooting and grace nurture one's cool-ing "yin" aspect which will balance the fire "yang" excess energies that the external styles of karate or "kung-fu" often build up to an excess in the body thus leading to premature inflammation, ageing and typical hard style illnesses.

Some of my training (clinical and martial art) was in Fujian province, which is historically notable not only as being the source of karate for Okinawa (and thus Japan) but also the main source of millions of Chinese immigrants to the States post WWII. Many Okinawans trained in Fujian while avoiding the mainland Japanese draft and oppression during the late 1800s and then later returned (often posing as Chinese) to Okinawa. Some of these returnees eventually taught some of the martial arts nowadays known as various karate styles. Some of the more well-known karate styles are Uechi-ryu, Shito-ryu, Goju-ryu, and Shoto-kan.

My favorite "sifu" (Chinese martial arts teacher), Master Jin, who had calluses on his wrists from striking with them over the years, always emphasized maximum forced breathing which one cannot do unless one is strong and has built up considerable internal "chi"/energy. Interestingly, he was born in the "Year of the Earth Rabbit" as was my favorite Japanese karate Sensei (Master Uehara). They were also both of similar physical stature being short, muscular and exceptionally strong. I trained with Master Jin at a live-in school for children training in martial arts in Fujian, China. This martial art school was run by a Ms. Wu, who aside from being highly trained and a kung-fu movie star, was the only woman allowed to run a "wushu" (kung-fu) school in China (I was told this by Mr. Li, Secretary General of the Fuken-sho Wushu Association who had hosted my clinical training and participation in the 1995 All China Wushu (kungfu) Competition). Ms.Wu was a lively, physically strong, energetic lady who enjoyed training. It was interesting that even these exceptional children, specially chosen and trained in many styles, would usually just end up going back to their hometown and teaching other children after they graduated. This perpetuates a large supply of martial artists all over the country. There is usually little of the romantic vision commonly associated in the West with martial arts among Chinese themselves.

Many of the health clinicians I have seen in various countries, despite their intelligence and other healing skills, lacked a developed sense of "chi" energy, as they had not trained properly for many years in any of the martial or yogic arts. In the States, in particular, many practitioners lack what I see as a developed sense of "chi" in both its practical application and clinical manipulation. This "command of chi" is often approximated by sincere but less experienced practitioners. It is a long-term process of gradual accumulation of "chi" which demands perseverance and an understanding of its significance. Most (there are exceptions) acupuncture colleges in the States offer merely a course or two in one style of martial art that is highly inadequate for chi development and understanding, as many years of proper training are necessary. As always, an experienced well-trained intuitive practitioner of any healing style can be very effective, but without a developed sense of "chi", they will be limiting themselves.

In **Fujian,** one sees an economic explosion largely funded by overseas remittances and Taiwanese investment. (Taiwan is just 135 miles across the strait.) Many Western companies now use partnerships with Taiwanese companies to more easily penetrate the Mainland Chinese market. (Mainland China has overtaken the States as Taiwan's largest export market). I was fortunate to be able to stay at a new condominium building being constructed by the family of one of my Taiwanese friends. This Taiwanese lady was also studying at the Traditional Chinese Medical University in Fuzhou although she was not sure if she really wanted to be a Doctor of Oriental Medicine back in Taiwan. However, as her family was successful, the doctor title respected, and she had a nice place to stay — why not. I saw this pattern with other intelligent financially supported Taiwanese who studied in Fuzhou because it was a convenient, close, inexpensive place to go to study while trying to figure out what one wanted to do with one's life.

While it was interesting and understandable to see the disdain between the Chinese and Japanese people in Tokyo, it was surprising and saddening to see the antipathy between the richer more educated Taiwanese Chinese and the local Fujian Chinese people. In the university/hospitals where I trained, the local Fujians were housed four to a simple room while the Taiwanese rented nicer local apartments. They did not socialize at all. Many Taiwanese considered the locals unrefined and poor. However, the locals knew the Taiwanese only studied in Fujian because they either could not get into or could not afford a Taiwanese medical school. The local Fujianese also wanted all the benefits of Taiwanese investment. A mutual type of need mixed with resentment seemed to prevail. The way they differed in thinking due to their exposure to ideas growing up made them more akin to foreigners than fellow Chinese. Both groups spoke Mandarin Chinese and most of the Taiwanese I met also spoke the local Fukenese dialect.

Personally, most Chinese people whom I met spoke Taiwanese or Fukenese, and treated me very kindly and friendly. As there are few Westerners in Fujian compared to the numbers in Guangzhou (Canton), Shanghai, or Beijing, I stood out more and received special attention (which was usually appreciated). In addition, as Fuzhou and Xiamen are more lucrative cities, it was an easier and safer place to acclimate oneself to China without all the overwhelming bustle and confusion of a Shanghai. Nevertheless, getting around in China alone is very hectic and challenging when not being fluent in the local Chinese dialect or Mandarin. (A great unifying feature in Chinese history is the fact that there is only one written Chinese language. Chinese can read the same script in different dialects. Mandarin is the national and ubiquitous "dialect".)

Oriental medical training in China usually requires more years than either Japan or the States. One may also incorporate Western medical training and practice both Western and Oriental medicine. One may also just study Oriental medicine, but the emphasis is on herbology over acupuncture by about sixty per-cent to fourty percent. Again, to my knowledge, they did not teach any of the wonderful Japanese techniques in the Chinese schools, but some teachers and students are aware of them and a few do study them on their own.

There were stories from the many Chinese doctors who had worked in Africa over the years under very difficult conditions of war and limited supplies (China particularly fostered post WWII diplomatic relations with Africa over the years and there are many exchange programs). Many of the older Chinese doctors had survived similarly trying experiences in China itself.

I have many poignant memories as the vacant look of elderly relatives waiting to wheel out their family member after major surgery (many stomach removals with up to ninety per-cent of the stomach being removed. The high stomach cancer in China (and Japan) is largely attributed to their excess use of salt and fire-cooked/smoked foods). There were no support staff, no nurses, and the relative or friend would wheel the post-operation table to a room bare save for an old bed and an I.V. stand. I particularly remember viewing my first tonsillectomy in China. It was between thoracic surgeries and one of the younger doctors motioned for me to come with him. He took me to a small dimly-lit room where a young female patient was sitting alone in a chair. The doctor proceeded to remove the tonsils with just a local ineffective anesthetic while the patient was sitting in the chair holding a bowl to catch her own blood. She did well not to gag too much and walked out after the procedure was over. Again, no antibiotics were used or particularly necessary; this was another example of Chinese strength and practicality.

China, being so isolated and ancient, also offers one a wonderful chance to see things from a new perspective. What a fresh way to reconsider one's paradigms and habitual stale thought processes which slowly imbue so many as people grow older and tend to stagnate in an overly familiar environment devoid of stimulating life changing impulses on a regular basis! The feisty, emotional, demonstrative and often naive Chinese opened my eyes to another way of life and attitude that I had not experienced before.

(The **Chinese Snakehead** phenomenon is worthy of note as it is often in the news and the fastest growing Chinese organized human smuggling organization in Asia at present. The criminal group is a household name throughout Asia, and law enforcement in the States and Europe has been dealing with them for years. They appear to be getting stronger and as I saw so often when I was living in Fujian, they were protected as many locals referred to them as an employment agency. Some smaller towns have lost all their men of working age to the lure of overseas income. In Fuzhou, the capital city of Fujian, there was no shortage of young men as they constantly streamed in from the surrounding areas to find work in this bustling city. Construction work seemed to be going on everywhere. I was approached in Japan and China about participating in some business ventures to help liberate Chinese from the mainland. Fortunately, I was able to gracefully avoid having to do anything illegal and still maintain my contacts and acquaintances.

I met many who proudly displayed items and lifestyles made possible by remittances from children living overseas. Despite the many media stories of average minimum fees of US$25,000, abuse and death of those being smuggled, the demand for the Snakehead's services to smuggle Chinese overseas remained robust. My impression from talking to so many families in Fujian was that there was no choice but to support the smugglers as the potential returns were lucrative and many parents and children alike felt that compared to a life in China, it was well worth risking some likely abuse.

As an example of the huge increase in numbers of **illegals,** a BBC documentary in 2001 stated that some 40,000 Chinese "tourists" flew into Yugoslavia, a known stepping-stone on the way to Western Europe, in 2000. Before that, the average was 300-400 a year. During the 1990s, increasing numbers were being smuggled through Guam to the States and through Russia to Western Europe.)

During my martial art training, I spent much time on various body pounding practices in two man teams. This "pounding" is called "gin jong jaw" ("iron-bell") or in Japanese **"kotei-kitae"** ("body-pounding"). This practice starts with light hitting (or slapping for young children). As one's strength builds and one's tendons are raised and become full as they absorb more "chi" one can tolerate increasingly forceful pounding. A slow individual process is involved that the student determines at his own pace. One makes quick progress if formally training three times a week with others. Daily pounding training is too tiring as the body needs time to rest and recuperate after proper training if it involves much physical contact. Incredible strength in taking a blow as well as striking and blocking are all imparted in these drills. Light contact training and other training is better daily. The initial emphasis is on the forearms, legs and stomach as these body parts are the most struck in training.

I have trained with some men who took full blows to their throat and groin (by voluntarily retracting the gonads with the cremaster muscle as sometimes occurs in very young boys involuntarily. It is interesting to actually see this retraction as many would think there is no place into which the testicles can withdraw). As one becomes more conditioned over the years, increased levels of concentration are necessary, for a momentary lapse in the proper concentration of energy at the point of impact i.e., where one will receive the blow on the body, can easily result in injury. I have had many bones fractured (but not broken) over the years from high impact blows and inadequate concentration on my part. I learned to distinguish the sensation of a blow that, for example, had fractured one of my bones from a blow that would merely cause a painful bruise. Likewise, I learned to sense which of my strikes was penetrating another's body deeply or not. These are very interesting distinctions to be able to perceive. This practice may sound abusive or sadistic to some people in this modern age, but it really is just part of the process of connecting to oneself at a deeper level physically. Another example of pain related therapy is in learning to deal with certain types of pain as a learning experience without taking medication for a while before actually healing the cause of the pain (as opposed to quickly taking pain reducing drugs as a knee jerk reaction to the first inkling of a muscular ache without asking what the pain could possibly signify at a deeper emotional level). Major injuries are not common. The striking individual at times can withdraw at the last second some of the power or intent of the strike if he believes it will injure the other. This refined sense must be acquired through trial and error. This style of training is an example of reestablishing contact with the instinctive "animal-self" that can lead to a heightened sense of awareness in other areas of life as well.

At the esoteric level, which is not traditionally taught until the student reaches a certain level, the practice of various two-man pounding exercises are direct **bone marrow stimulus** and abdominal organ massage. These drills are believed by many Buddhists and Taoists to stimulate healthier blood cell production as well as keep the marrow full and the bones strong so that the usual degradation of the marrow portion of the marrow producing bones (femur, ribs etc...) does not occur as much. Normally the percentage of the bone occupied by marrow decreases a little as one gets older and the quality of the blood cells produced is generally thought to be less potent. This results in less vitality in many ways. This pounding training may seem crude to some but it is very effective judging from the vitality of many such practitioners and teachers that I have known over many years.

We are taught in martial arts, yoga and Oriental medical schools that different body parts can hold different amounts of "chi" energy. The fascia (connective tissue running throughout the whole body) seems to be able to absorb large amounts of "chi" which can be used or stored in reserve. The "chi-hai" point CV6 (1.5 "cun" (inch) below the umbilicus) is thought to be the main energy "chi" accumulation point in the body and thus the emphasis on abdominal training and proper Buddhist "jeng hu shi" or Taoist "reverse" breathing "faan hu shi" techniques (empirically, Tibetan techniques seem to provide quicker results). Abdominal massage and later stomach pounding will build the energy here quickly. The ability to withstand stomach pounding is generally used as a reflection of how much "chi" energy the person has accumulated thus the pride of being able to take a full punch in the stomach. Once the "chi" has been built up enough at this abdominal "chi hai" point it can then be distributed around the torso "sheau jou tian" (small circulation) and eventually out to the limbs "da jou tian" (grand circulation).

Cultivating one's own "chi" in the abdominal area allows for a different important type of sensitivity in diagnosing the imbalances of others when touching a patient's abdominal area ("hukushin") as is emphasized in Japanese acupuncture and healing. Many people in metaphysics also realize that the Oriental chakras can be different in the abdominal area. The abdominal centre **("hara"** in Japanese) is a seat of both energy and emotion within the body that the Japanese emphasize greatly in their culture. This is evidenced by the many idioms in the Japanese language that refer to the abdomen as a center for emotion. There are also some idiomatic expressions in many languages such as in the American English terms, "He has guts" or "spilling one's guts". Some examples in Japanese are: "hara guroi"- (black guts) scheming or black hearted "hara no mushi"- (stomach insect) one's mood or feeling "hara o waru"- (split open one's guts) show one's true feeling "hara o kimeru"- (decide one's stomach) be resolved to do something

Proper breathing techniques i.e., techniques involving the anal/vaginal sphincter closure "bih gang" that have been known for ages must become more widely taught in the States. I was saddened upon returning to the States that so few yogic teachers, martial

artists and physicians even knew about the significance of the anal/
vaginal sphincter balancing. So many practitioners are teaching insufficient superficial deep breathing techniques and thus denying
many of the simple and powerful balancing treatment.

Over the years, I have seen that there is at times a breaking
of the rhythmic cycle of chi circulation that prevents energy from
getting up high enough in the body. This breaking seems to relate
to the rhythmic contraction of **sphincter muscles** in the large
intestine, and these muscles present in diaphragm in their relationship to the mouth and anus/vagina do both appear to be of critical
importance in their timing. This aspect is a purely physical, but
must be understood to be able to best move these energies, because
an individual cannot be the one to choose where that energy is
best utilized — sometimes for thinking or the brain, other times
it is best when put into the arms and shoulders or other times into
the heart for emotional expression as well as improved circulation.
Amazingly the body seems to naturally integrate and balance when
the sphincters timing and breath techniques is a coordinated activity. Thus, the appropriate synchronization of these muscles does
provide good health long term.

Another area of tapping stimulation is the sternum. This tapping can be done forcefully with developed fingertips or knuck-
les and this reverberates to the master immune endocrine gland
called the thymus. The **thymus** (and the pineal) have been the
lesser known of the seven endocrine glands among patients over
the years. The thymus sits behind the upper part of the sternum
and is soft pinkish gray lymph tissue shaped like a butterfly. This
gland is largest in youth and degrades after puberty, and is very
small in adults. It secretes hormones such as thymosin, serum
thymic factor and

thymopoetin which balance the immune response especially cell-mediated immunity (cell immunity not regulated by antibodies). Low levels of these hormones in the blood are associated with lowered immune balancing capabilities. The December 13, 2001 issue of Nature reported the regeneration of thymus from thymic epithelial cells. However, in metaphysical clinics certain "subtle energy" devices (such as specific gauss polarity magnets, crystals, lasers, inert gas devises) and eating aged raw thymus have been found to regenerate its function. However, it is best for parents to teach the children to keep their own thymus stimulated with tapping games that the child can continue doing for life if trained from a young age. The important thing to remember is that when working with different body parts, aside from increasing the functionality of the physical body part, increasing the energy interchange between the "etheric subtle body"* and the physical body is key. The thymus stimulus is essential here as it is an important gateway that is associated with various chakras* and glands.

*In metaphysical literature the human body is usually divided into 7-12 subtle "layers" of a more "etheric" nature which lie outside of our physical body. These **subtle bodies** relate to how we receive energy from the higher aspects of our soul and spirit. Dr. Rudolph Steiner's Anthroposophical Approach to Medicine Anthroposophical Press. 1957

*Chakras** are considered to be energy vortices in our "subtle bodies" that connect with the physical body and adjust higher vibrational energies. There are seven main chakras that relate to our seven main endocrine glands and their related organs. Hundreds of smaller chakras as seen to be the main acupuncture points. Alice Bailey, Esoteric Healing N.Y. Lucis Publishing 1980

Martial Arts, Meditation and Brain Coherence

Martial-arts training helps one reconnect with the animal instincts inherent in all humans. Repeated motions, such as blocks and strikes, eventually become instinctive. One can react without the interference of the slower process of thinking. One also learns to draw on the group energy. In various Asian training halls I would initially struggle with language impediments trying to understand different techniques or moves intellectually. Eventually, I realized that words were often not necessary. I learned to watch others' martial art movements more carefully and actually feel others' movements as well as my own movements more over the years. Thus, many times I felt it was a definite advantage to train without clear explanations and translations. Some martial art teachers do not verbally explain much in accordance with Zen tradition. This is just an example of many types of instinctive non-verbal training that leads one back to Mother Earth and the source of much of human energy inherent in oneself.

The ability to move energy, to see it shared, is an important attribute that is not that well developed amongst clinical healers, acupuncturists, massage therapists etc.., because they are doing it physically with their hands or needles. Many alternative healers/ workers are deficient in this ability because they do not have sufficient connection to the natural world. The phenomenon of energy has certain attributes that are frictional for people as they reach a threshold with it. Martial Arts can move energy and help people attune to this.

In the brain is the source of the manifestation of every aspect of the body. It is the source of expression for the growing consciousness that shapes and forms everything. Spirit manifests through the brain in the creation of thought and ideas and many other energies that shape our physicality. **That is to say that the source of human intelligence is not local. It is as though the brain were a transformer of incoming energies that over evolution have shaped it physically in order to adapt human consciousness.** This is a core or source of life force that is available and can be transferred. The Chinese understood this idea of the brain as source, and this is one of the reasons they called the brain the "sea of bone marrow". A certain transfer of energy from the brain comes more through vibrational levels than the physical so the consciousness associated with any movement of energy is more important than the physical action of the brain. **However, the available level of this coherent energy available in the brain is rarely accessed.** Most individuals thought patterns relate back to random nerve firings that are largely incoherent. **Neurons releasing/firing together equals coherency and this allows for magnetic field fluctuations to be in resonance and as a result much stronger** (it may help to think of coherency as a laser beam as opposed to a regular flashlight). In the brain this is called linear coherence as opposed to coherence as measured in the heart. The heart is rhythmical. One can consider popular music to see how different the musical/brain forms are from the rhythmical/heart sounds and yet how beautiful they combine. In their alignment and coherency, which is a much higher level of Martial Arts practice, all kinds of powerful energies are available simply because of the density of neurons. Many of these neurons seem to create electrical patterns and then in a coherent manner create magnetic patterns. These magnetic patterns have effect at a distance in the world, in one's body and the bodies of others. This is an alternate scientific way of utilizing more modern understanding to explain this but, inherently understood by the Chinese as opportunity for all kinds of energies as pure source. The potential here is tremendous.

Meditation is a step in the direction of coherency but, there is much more to it than that. Indeed, meditation can be that which involves only a small portion of the brain at any given time. The activation of many brain components simultaneously is truly a martial arts practice just as when one is doing some martial art form or "kata" moving and focusing on one part of the body; it is how one starts. But, as one gets better at it, the same movement might even appear to someone else as the same movement with which one began. It changes for one because there is far more awareness of every aspect of the body. When one is focusing on movement of the hands, one becomes more aware of the feet and how every aspect of the body is positioned. Why should this awareness stop there? Why not extend this also to the brain and the activity that it is involved in. A tremendous amount of constant activity in the brain is autonomic and governs all of the attributes of the rest of your body. All this must be available as the neurons are all in the same approximation. They are all close to each other and can share energy if you use it. **Some would not do so fearing that perhaps they would damage the body by turning that which is autonomic into something that which might, under their conscious control, cause them harm.** At first thought that is an understandable concern. However, this is the same sort of energy that is understood in regards to martial arts practice where you take any aspect or function and make it more conscious. The combining of the disciplines of meditation and martial arts continues to hold great promise. There is a natural rhythm associated with brain wave function close to the Schumann resonance frequency of the earth (which averages around eight cycles per second) which is able to work at harmonic submultiples of this clustered in the delta region frequencies.

The standing waves represent several frequencies with the fundamental one being 7.8 Hz. I assume that the Schumann average will increase. The opportunities to work with these energies are rarely used by individuals in a conscious state because one would usually be half-asleep and eventually fall asleep or wake up. Typically the meditations might involve tapes, mantras etc...but, as one goes deeper with this, there is a natural sense of merging, becoming one with all things. Under such circumstances, the continuation of the meditation is difficult to continue in any conscious sense because one would seem to be directing it, implying separation of the director and that which is directed and yet in the oneness the energies are all present. This experience is one of the beginning of coherency throughout the brain. The capacity to produce this coherence is simply that of these brainwave states being natural, with which one easily accesses and works.

The brain naturally goes through these frequencies all day and night, so it is nothing that the person has to create. Hence, the understanding of this at a technological level can be provided to some extent by biofeedback and techniques utilized to enhance theta brainwave states. Martial arts are one method of sharing energy throughout the entire physical body. Eventually, as in so many things of this nature, it is a rediscovery of naturally occurring aspects that are already present.

To do martial art training in the lower frequencies is desirable for those who are looking for special training not commonly done. As one moves through the Alpha frequencies, one eventually comes into the Delta range. One can easily sense the shift in brain wave patterns without actually measuring them. It is very difficult for most individuals to work with these lower frequencies during any physical body movement as one would fall down or be sleeping but the masters have indeed learned this and by their example this can be taught.

HEALING FOR HEALING'S SAKE

"And even in our sleep pain that cannot forget falls drop by drop upon the heart, and in our own despair, against our will, comes wisdom by the awful grace of God." Aeschylus (one translation from Agamemnon)

I have been fortunate to have worked in so many different clinical settings over the years, which have led to better understanding, knowledge and insight as to how to help and approach patients. In hindsight, I regret how comparatively little I could offer patients at my first acupuncture clinic. I have often thought how great it would be to retreat certain patients now that I think that I have so much more to offer them.

The various approaches I have had to determine what is best for a patient have led to a new awareness of how to properly integrate various empirical and academic knowledge. What usually arises is the same aspect of integration that is being required in all areas of medical science i.e., education. The patient is self-empowered, shown how to move the energies him or herself, how to learn about the proper texts to read, proper ways to understand and work with this new energy and knowledge. Indeed, the more the energy is concentrated in the hands of the teacher or acupunctourist as the authority, the more difficulties will inevitably ensue. Understanding this larger principal is much more than particular techniques or practices — it is an awareness of much longer-term energies whereby which some patients come up with new methods and new understandings to share that will in a future time (even a future reincarnation) be very useful.

I always have interesting material for patients to read in the English, Chinese and Japanese languages. Many patients get discouraged with various readings but those that continue to inquire, study and/or experiment make great strides in mind and body. The challenge for me over the years has been deciding how much information and of what nature to discuss with patients. Some patients with limited spiritual, medical or metaphysical knowledge are easily intimidated or raise an eyebrow at new information that is outside their personal realm of consciousness. The healer or friend must use intuition or experience to know what specific information with which to tease that person to arouse curiosity and excitement about new ways to consider health, body or emotional makeup. There is usually some way to reach most people that come to a metaphysically oriented clinic. Sometimes that window is small or the information may be basic but for that person it is the right place to begin and hopefully later they can integrate and eventually manifest it in the future. **Accessibility, acceptability, absorbability and integration must be considered carefully for each person.**

To engage the inquiry process within my own consciousness has always been a natural thing for me to do: asking myself why I did this and why others do what they do. In my meditations, I have always enjoyed reliving intense, wonderful or thoughtless experiences in my life to refeel the emotions I experienced then.

As all the emotions one ever feels are imprinted on one's astral body, it is just a matter of what I call "sucking" these vibrations a bit closer to my physical body to allow them to reconnect with my consciousness — almost like a video replay. **It is similar to how real some "dreams" seem upon awakening.** Emotions, particularly those accumulated from birth, tend to clog up the web of energy around people. It is a practical idea to relive events in a nonjudgmental way and then sever that string of the web to become more karmically independent. **However, to stimulate this inquiry process in others is quite an art.** After many years of ups and downs in terms of help-ing patients deal with the root causes of their imbalances and the thought processes involved, I saw that my questions had been too difficult and devoid of sufficient compassion and caring. Therefore, the individual received the harder edge rather than the process of inquiry ignited in themselves. When I finally realized that the real benefit regarding questions that engage the receiver was a psycho-logical one, I no longer had to look for the truth. Up until that time, I had relied on two types of inquiry processes to find the truth. One was in myself, asking myself questions and looking at my own beliefs, breaking down my own understanding and bring-ing greater clarification to myself. The other was in the world of objective facts, realities and experiments. As I became more expe-rienced, I was able to engage intuition and utilize subtle energies as well as overt physics and various widely available technologies that all proved comprehensive and effective. However, I finally realized that none of this had anything to do with the inquiry process ignited in others.

The real point is to begin a resonant principal. It is similar to how "Tai Chi Chuan" ("Great Ultimate Fist" the most widely known of the three internal martial art styles, the other two being

"Hsing-yi" and "Ba-Kua") is taught by the masters. It is as if a sort of jump-start transfers the energy from the healer, the teacher, the other into the recipient with the correct direction that the person will have to continue the process. So then can the inquiry process be fun and engaging. **In generating the right series of questions for another person to ask, there can be so much caring and sincerity that the individual then is able to love oneself even when the an-swers that show up are those that are very difficult for the person to hear.** The answers to questions might generate shame, guilt or struggle inside the person. The answer might generate some aspect that the person wants to resist, deny or rebel against, but if there is enough love and caring perhaps jump-started by the healer's energy, they will continue inquiring instead of attaching. People tend to be in either of these two conditions-inquiring or attaching. If you are attaching, you will be working with energies you have al-ready built on as an experiment, as an experience, as a belief struc-ture. All these energies can have value but by and large, you will not receive the value because you are attaching and not inquiring. As humans we must develop a way of speaking to others that really reaches them; a way in which the manifestation of the full nature of the being, the love that we all have inside ourselves, the motivation that brings us to want to heal/help and make a difference. It is not just about money or even seeing that people get better. It's not just about contributing.

There is another aspect to it — the aspect that heals for healing's sake, or in a larger sense, the energy that loves for love's sake. Gradually the unconditional human love emerges through that inquiry process and when that is given to another as a question is asked, even a very difficult question that makes someone look deeply into themselves, changes are profound. If the jump-start is sufficient, they will continue the inquiry process, which will be far more powerful and effective than anything we as healers or teachers could do for them directly. As healer/ teacher/human, to feel this love flow right through oneself is actually wonderful and deeply pleasurable — more than many might imagine.

I have known people in more than a dozen countries on four continents from all walks of life. I saw that what was lacking in some of them, as in myself, was that despite having various levels of truth, happiness, life experience and wealth, there was still a hollowness because that which was missing, this truly unique aspect of love and compassion, was difficult to actually apply effectively in life. **It is this need to apply, as opposed to the mere perception of the existence of this aspect of compassion, that sits in some peoples' subconscious and slowly redirects their lives as they raise their level of awareness enough to access, accept, absorb, and perhaps integrate "new" radical ideas and knowledge** — much of which has been available or soon will be.

In the development of consciousness there seems to exist a path of clarification and evolution, a need to assist, for most people. Through assistance, one can learn a great deal about other people, about themselves. The "universal law of reflection" is able to work more consciously as one understands this law and can play with such energies. Many involved in the healing arts work in this arena and as they move through the various levels, they begin to recognize such capacities as the healing of the soul etc...

Many healers will then begin to notice within themselves greater excitement as well as a greater sense of responsibility to appropriately apply the healing providing hints that this healing path is continuing to be challenging, exciting and interesting. When they reach such levels, some people, often move away from the healing professions finding instead that other things draw their attention, having thus completed this particular path of assistance. As one moves through any path of assistance, one begins to recognize that through the assistance is developed a sense-of-self, a sense of awareness, a deeper understanding and capacity to interrelate to various components within oneself. One is able to make more rapid spiritual progress and evolve many aspects of consciousness by the utilization of the principal of assistance.

Healing is a subset of the path of assistance. There are many ways to assist others in life but "true" assistance i.e. evolution and clarification, involves allowing for a shift at the higher energy/ vibrational levels. Clarification does not come only from mental understanding. Indeed, **the mental energies sometimes block the higher levels of healing because these energies are powerfully associated with old habit patterns, thought forms of a destructive nature or other aspects**. What I feel one can learn by healing for healing's sake is the path by which the assistance that one allows is seen as an important component of all human life — aspects related to the law of love and the law of human health as they then relate to one's own consciousness, the law of reflection. The result of this is greater attunement and affinity to the healing energies and the awareness of the healing principal at all levels. This attunement can have the effect of completing, but it can also have the effect of opening and allowing whole new areas of not only technology and healing but a new attitude of understanding and awareness. For this reason some people follow the healing path specifically to balance "karma" to attune for or balance for those they have harmed in the past. In doing so there can be a completion to part of this life cycle and a new path begun, or it can lead one to a deeper understanding of the healing process as an important form of the entire study of existentiality.

To assist and to understand what assisting is about is a complex matter. To a large extent, it involves a significant component that is very direct, is very physical, that which is felt in the consciousness more than it is simply intelligence or utilization of **cosmo-ethic principals** or interrelationship having to do with technology. This direct attunement to consciousness is a difficult matter to explain but that which everyone to some extent can feel in basic energy touching therapies, such as massage, that allow one to feel a sense of upliftment, a sense of peace, a sense of something bigger than oneself, even a hint of love or its source. This 'sensation" is the most basic aspect of existentiality because it does not necessarily involve the thought process. This is a positive useful experience for everyone and that which is felt at physical as well as non-physical levels.

PART II: DIET (RAW VS. COOKED)

ALL RAW FOOD REFERENCES REFERS TO ORGANIC OR NATURALLY GROWN OR RAISED FOODS (meat, fat, fruit, vegetables etc)

My first dramatic introduction to raw food for healing was as a nineteen-year old living in southern Spain. I had been camping outside and hitchhiking heading south on my way to Morocco and had come down with something like pneumonia. I was sleeping in isolated orchards in between towns and some gypsies had taken me in on their way to one of the well-known horse shows in Sevilla. A beautiful dark featured lady with a commanding presence had given me something to drink which I thought tasted particularly good in my delirious state; I later found out the drink was raw goat milk mixed with fresh goat blood. I still remember this truly enchanting lady whom I knew as Mercedes who encouraged me to keep sipping on my drink seemingly every few minutes. She would methodically whisper in my ear, "Siempre hay una sonrisa en el ojo de la mente." ("There is always a smile in the eye of the mind") which is a phrase that I would come back to many times in my life.

It would be many years later before I researched the true value of raw dairy, raw foods, raw meat and microbes and their essential role in healing. Raw foods have become a main part of my clinical practice and have allowed for the deepest healing and rebuilding I have ever seen in my clients. It is very satisfying to help people heal themselves naturally through diet and become more consciously in control of their lives at such an intimate level.

Many people will learn to become their own initial health consultant after they become familiar with the raw foods and do basic research. This way of thinking allows for a greatly decreased sense of dependency on the mainstream "medical/pharmaceutical/insurance community" which has in many ways undermined society's development and healthcare.

While living in Asia during the 1990s, I found people were more aware of the benefits of raw foods and healthful bacteria and were not as exposed to erroneous fear-based perspectives as sponsored by Western media. Thus Asians stayed more connected with their basic instincts and were more suspicious of medicine that Westerners gulp down so naively or desperately. I remember offering a Japanese friend an aspirin for a headache once and being surprised by her sincere very concerned response that she does not take medicine. I repeated that it was just aspirin, but her explanation revealed that in her thinking medicine is medicine and it is not good for the body except in an emergency. She did not distinguish between aspirin and stronger pain medicine available with or without a prescription. Her seemingly simplistic way of thinking impressed me very much, as I had grown up in a Western medical household and had become familiar with the common use and prescriptions of muscle relaxants, pain pills and antibiotics. I would often use antibiotics at the first sign of a sore throat or cold. My Japanese friend's surprising response about what was to me a common, weak and safe pill like aspirin had pleasantly aroused my undermined instincts. Over the years, I would question many people in various Asian countries to try to understand their unadulterated thinking about medicine. I learned much that has been of value to me.

An example of Japanese natural diet habits is their ingestion of various raw seafood and fermented high bacteria soybean paste called "natto." These are two very popular, healthful foods that provide raw fats, raw protein and many useful healing bacteria strains. Many Westerners fortunately are learning the benefits of clean wild raw seafood, but few can stand the strong bacteria smell or taste of bacterial foods such as "natto." (In conversation, Japanese like to challenge foreigners by asking if they can eat "natto.") Increasing number of healthful drinks, as well as bacteria-based products, was also available on the Japanese market such as Dr. Teruo Higa's "Effective Microorganism (EM)" products that can be modified for enhanced health.

The natural organic diet is largely raw fat and raw protein based. Overwhelming scientific evidence exists clearly showing that raw fats naturally draw out many toxins and rebuild the nervous system, some hormones and cellular wall structure, which are well-known to be high in lipids. Raw animal fats have interesting unique building properties in the human body, and the fruit fats have cleansing properties. Raw dairy, such as milk, butter, cheese and cream, are also essential for both rapid healing and rebuilding. Raw dairy often needs to be purchased from a local farm or ordered over the Internet. Avocado, oils, coconut, seeds, nuts and fruits are also important depending upon the detoxifying or rebuilding venue. An important basic of the diet is "balancing" the various body pH (hydrogen potential) systems (not just blood pH) by adjusting acidic and alkaline foods. A rule of thumb is the more acidic raw meats and organs at one meal must be balanced with the more alkalinizing raw vegetable juice at another meal. The body's pH systems actually can not really be changed much as the body has many buffer systems to prevent such. Changing quickly from acidic to alkaline and back is refreshing to the body.

These buffer systems are what really become challenged and strained as they maintain the various system pH within a strict narrow range. If the pH is too alkalin, one would die. Most people tend to be a spec more acidic than is ideal. If I sense an acidic feeling, I will just drink some fresh squeezed lemon as it has the most alkalinizing effect.

Hopefully, one eventually can learn to prepare food on which one has cultivated bacteria to produce stronger and deeper healing and rebuilding i.e., high meats. In Asia I often had drinks prepared with aged-fish. The fish were aged for a couple of weeks while being aired to allow many strains of useful healing aerobic bacteria to grow on the fish. These drinks and other aged foods conferred strong feelings of happiness but tasted awful.

The sense of well-being that aged high bacteria food imparts to humans is due to the bacterias direct production of feel good hormones/neurotransmitters like dopamine and serotonin and interaction with chromaffin cells in the small intestine.

Most of the serotonin is produced in the the small intestine where it influences peristalsis (natural intestinal movement). One can start by trying an easy aspect of the diet such as raw coconut cream or vegetable juicing. Then, due to feeling better in some way, one is encouraged to try other phases of the diet such as natural raw eggs or a bite of organic/natural raw ground beef or even bacon (which tastes good).

It has been very interesting seeing how patients adopt different parts of the Primal-raw food diets. A main difficulty I have found has been dispelling understandable but erroneous fear of bacteria from raw sources of naturally raised meats, dairy, and foods cultivated for bacterial growth sometimes called "high meats." Another impediment is the common dislike of certain textures. The main overall problem for many people is understanding the undermining need for "good tasting/smelling" food. The energy expenditure of most people over deciding many times daily what to eat, where to eat, whom to meet for coffee etc...is a great distraction and needs to be reconsidered and redirected. A cultural example is the popular Japanese fermented soy-bean paste called "natto," which is previously mentioned. This paste is very popular with Japanese children and adults and yet has a very strong offensive smell to most non-Japanese. It is sold in small single-serving packets in Asian markets all over the world and has a high bacteria count that many ingest frequently for health and enjoyment. Westerners especially find the smell very strong and offensive. This is an excellent example of culturally based sense determination i.e., many Japanese say it tastes and smells good or not bad. Most Westerners I know find it very "gross" in smell and most refuse to even try it.

Interestingly, many of my Japanese clients who love "natto" (and also eat raw fish, raw eggs, and many different unique-tasting Japanese foods) refuse to eat a small dime-size piece of an aged-meat that even they agree does not smell as strong as natto. Again, the natto is many bites of a chewy moist "smelly" substance, and the aged meat is a tiny piece of harder dry meat (even fish) that can be swallowed without chewing and so there need not be any taste. This is an example of programming one's brain/senses and an indication of what can be done consciously to reprogram ones thinking and senses. Reprogramming consciously is also a fun experiment for oneself.

Increasingly people will see the necessity and practicality of eating raw organic, natural food and a high raw fat diet to both limit toxin intake and effectively draw-out accumulated heavy metals and neurotoxins which are known to be raw fat soluble (Aschner et al 1990). Of course, healing and a sense of happiness are quicker to come from the small intestine, which produces many healing and "feel good" chemicals, if one also ingests aged-foods with many different bacteria strains. These raw diets have allowed many people to heal themselves and their children, as well as discover a new sense of empowerment and joy in life. A society, such as in the States, could benefit much from such a raw healthful diet, and the potential lowering of crime and drug-addiction rates to prescription drugs so readily used to alter brain chemicals to lower the consciousness level of our depressed, hyperactive, and sad. When the body's cornucopia of chemicals is fine tuned, largely through diet, people feel healthy and happy and many would be able to socially interact more harmoniously.

Getting people to switch to a raw food diet including raw meat and aged-meat is a unique challenge since the predominant wisdom, the "**consensus reality,**" exerts itself through an emotional tie. Thus, the individual will revert to his or her own feelings and these are completely out of proportion to the action involved relating to a few bacteria. <u>It is as if all the fear, all the energies associated with many of the activities of a fear-oriented media have made many feel impotent and afraid.</u> There are so many ways in which the illusions of life itself have been so deeply associated with bacteria at the level of psychology; it is often necessary to help them identify their fears and to look at them consciously. Still, many individuals will be best led by example. The fact that I can say that I use bacteria and aged meats on a regular basis despite being leery and it helped me anyway has given many patients the confidence to try it. (Empirically, it is obvious that depressed patients feel the most dramatic and rapid improvement from a high bacteria diet.) Many who object at seemingly scientific levels are actually speaking from fear. They are not speaking at all with regards to science because you can produce copious amounts of scientific wisdom and they will still be afraid. **The consensus reality has a strong hold on the masses and allows for a repression of the greatest healers, the greatest doctors on the planet i.e., bacteria.**

Now, when dealing with the fear issues, it is usually necessary to instill sufficient emotional response in the individual that they will then try something for themselves. When they find that they are not harmed and/or improved in health by that which they try, they can then reject some of the teachings of the consensus reality in the medical community and from this make their way to a deeper understanding. Each individual must find this path for him or herself. Any steps taken in this direction during this life, no matter how small, may allow for increased appreciation of resources available in the next life. The scientists who eventually embrace this principal will be able to design bacteria in the same way in which bacteria have been designed for warfare and destruction. Bacteria and viruses can be designed for healing and be of far greater effectiveness than anything currently available.

A fingertip of organic farm dirt is by far the cheapest quickest way to build bacteria . It must be remembered that if the underlying issues are of fear, it does no good to waste one's time trying to address issues with relationship to science. The new Ebola strains in the future will test most individuals and may well kill most of those infected.

A few individuals will understand bacteria, viruses and parasites in an intuitive way and do well with microbial ingestion or implantation without needing an explanation or research material to read. However, when trying to change someone's underlying reaction to some stimuli in the physical, it must be understood that these reactions are usually out of the individual's conscious control. The only way to change them is to show them how the recommended course of action is different from what they are doing or how it works for the healer. Again, the most dramatic results come from depressed patients who are so utterly miserable that they desperately try the high bacteria meats or soil as a last straw attempt and are pleasantly surprised. The regret and frustration is always that it took so many weeks, months or years of prodding before they reversed their depression with such a simple technique.

New energies and ideas are made available throughout the day when one consciously chooses not to be manipulated daily by the mass consciousness by following the marketing, advertising and erroneous research in so many areas of life. A new independence in life becomes available to enjoy. The individual becomes the researcher, the educator, the healer, the philosopher. One becomes more intuitive and becomes a better judge of information which one does receive. A great feeling of confidence and strength is gradually acquired.

I often tell my patients about the first time I was treated to "torahugu" (tiger blowfish sushi that is a winter delicacy in Japan). I knew that it was potentially poisonous, but as everyone was eating it, I assumed that it was perfectly safe. I would later learn that the blowfish tetrodotoxin can be 3,000 times more potent than mor-phine (good point) and 270 times more deadly than cyanide (bad point).(7) A few people still die yearly from ingesting improperly cleaned blowfish as sushi and a smaller species of blowfish is used to produce toxin induced voodoo zombie-like deaths in the Caribbean. Even eating the cleaned fish can give the sensation of tingling in the mouth. A homeopathic-type remedy of this drug (and many others) was used safely and effectively to facilitate certain stages of meditative practice among certain philosophical sects. Initially, it can be a scary thrill to feel the temporary physical paralysis while being mentally alert. The difference between a chemical being a toxic "poison" or an enhancing medicine has often been one of concentration of dosage and preparation.

(Again, I am not speaking of ingesting dangerous well-known pathogenic microorganisims that will sicken or kill humans.)

I have been in countries where during outbreaks of diarrhea (which sickens millions worldwide, kills millions, and is caused by many different organisms) the most effective and simple remedy we discovered was to simply filter the water through native clothing (acting as a filter). This will only work if the causative agent of the illness is big enough to be filtered out by the stitching size (which some bacteria as well as many worms, parasites and microorganisms are.)

SOME SCIENTIFIC FACTS
Evidence based health care will change the status quo.

Two thought provoking facts that I like to stress with patients are that there are many times more microbes in the human body than human cells, and that human nucleic DNA contains bacterial and fungal DNA sequences (Campbell and Reece, 2002). Having DNA sequences from bacteria, parasites, archaea, and fungus, affords humans great adaptive and survival abilities that have evolved for mutual benefit over eons. Bacteria, fungus, parasites, and arachaea are not foreign entities to humans. Humans have an ancient special evolutionary history with bacteria and other microbes. **Our body has an innate need and ability to work with microbes for the advancement of each other.** Humans can learn to consciously connect with and communicate with bacteria and even viruses to help direct the bacteria in healing and changing our bodies. **It is a symbiotic relationship evidenced in our DNA.** Pondering these facts can facilitate arriving at a new perspective of what it means to be "human" as well as what is logically part of a natural human diet. By slowly introducing new strains of bacteria into our diet, a direct communication can be developed which may influence the bacteria in its well known, scientifically verifiable, and proven ability to morph, share DNA with other bacteria via transformation, plasmids, pathogenicity islands and phages and even revert into more primordial forms like viruses, parts of which are well known to be able to enter human DNA. (Viruses are now used in medicine in many ways such as DNA/gene insertion, but some are already consciously creating these to evolve more quickly.

As an example of how misunderstood bacteria are let's use the well known *Escherichia coli (E-coli)* bacteria scares which are so commonly heard in the media as an example. Actually, there are now around 700 strains of *E-coli* of which just a few cause various illnesses: diarrhea, neonatal meningitis, and urinary tract infections in humans. *E. coli* is a consistent inhabitant of the human intestinal tract, and it is the predominant facultative organism in the human GI tract. It can live with or without oxygen (Clark et al., 2002). Therefore, when one hears that a quick preliminary test revealed *e-coli* in the public water it really means little until they identify which strain (this takes time). The odds of it being pathogenic are small.

E. coli has around 4000 genes. It can respond to environmental signals such as chemicals, pH, temperature, osmolarity, etc., in a number of very remarkable ways considering it is a unicellular organism. For example, it can sense the presence or absence of chemicals and gases in its environment and swim towards or away from them. Or it can stop swimming and grow fimbriae that will specifically attach it to a cell or surface receptor. In response to change in temperature and osmolarity, it can vary the pore diameter of its outer membrane porins to accommodate larger molecules (nutrients) or to exclude inhibitory substances. With its complex mechanisms for regulation of metabolism the bacterium can survey the chemical contents in its environment in advance of synthesizing any enzymes that metabolize these compounds. It does not wastefully produce enzymes for degradation of carbon sources unless they are available, and it does not produce enzymes for synthesis of metabolites if they are available as nutrients in the environment. Bacteria also produce various defenses against antibiotics and can share this genetic trait with other bacteria. (The Good, the Bad, and the Deadly *SCIENCE*- June 4, 2004)

The few pathogenic strains commonly cause minor intestinal and urinary problems which healthy people recover from soon often without medicine. Giving antibiotics for diarrhea caused by many intestinal bacteria may worsen the condition temporarily if the bacterial toxin is then released into the body in large amounts as the bacteria die. The few strains that are really pathogenic (like EHEC 0157: H7) are worrisome because they have absorbed or acquired special DNA via phages, plasmids, and pathogenicity islands that allow the bacterium to attach and efface the intestinal track wall, actually inject Shiga toxin via specialized secretion systems, secrete exotoxins that cause lysis of red blood cells, and express other putative virulence factors. Amazing for a one cell organism typically 3 microns long (three one-thousands of a millimeter) but with DNA more than 300 times longer.

I am promoting the idea that one can learn to influence one's own DNA through the inherent evolutionary link which exists between viruses and bacterial intelligence and human intelligence. It is naturally in all of us as a gift of evolution. **As viruses are not to be found on the tree of life one must logically consider that humans can make them consciously !**

Humans must learn to take the next step in consciousness healing and evolutionary promotion by reconnecting with an aspect of themselves that they have been taught to fear, demean and kill. This is another example of masochism and lack of self-love that powerful interests manipulate to undermine an individual's sense of self-control, self determination and increase one's sense of fear and impotence.

I have found that only a fingertip of organic soil from a farm has enough bacteria to heal rapidly- especially mental health. Various bacterial strains can either directly produce mood enhancing neurotransmitters/hormones like Serotonin and Dopamine or direct the brain to do so via peptides.

The most significant basic scientific health-related fact is that most cooked food is toxic. Although through time raw foods have been acknowledged as biologically healing, raw food diets will become predominant as man evolves to higher levels of consciousness. Raw foods allow for healing at the deepest (cellular) level, as opposed to the important, but mostly symptomatic relief provided most treatments. Today this raw natural human diet is known by names such as "Paleo" or "Primal" diet. It includes any raw food including fruits, dairy, meats, vegetables, organs and high bacteria foods. The key is to ingest sufficient amounts of raw proteins and raw fats to biologically and scientifically clean and rebuild the body from a cellular basis. I and other clinicians have found that ingested cooked food slows down the healing process. Overall, there are no unique benefits from complex carbs. This diet is an ancient traditional human diet still practiced by some today. I refer to it as a natural human diet.

A plethora of exists supporting the idea that high-heated/ cooked proteins, fats, and grains produce cytotoxins, mutagens and carcinogens:
heterocyclic amines (as in cooked meats)
lipid oxides(as in cooked fats)
acrylamides (as in baked breads and coffee) nitrosamines (as in tobacco and cooked fish); urethanes (in many foods like cooked dairy, soy, and bread), pthalates etc.. . (1-14)

- **I stress here that research (mostly Japanese and European but more recently the National Cancer Institute) shows that about 20 different mutagenic toxic heterocyclic amines (HA) can be formed by heating amino acids (in muscle meats) with creatine (also in muscle meat) during cooking.**

Research is very detailed and specific as there are different types of DNA mutations that are at present more implicated in activating oncogenes i.e., transversions. The natural DNA repair mechanisms are varied and fascinating so each cell can often over-come/ repair common mutations or even trigger apoptosis- cellular suicide to protect the body. In one research study, 75% of mutations induced in hamster ovary cells by a HA were transversions (Yuan et al. 1994); as opposed to the 95% frameshift mutations induced by 9 different HAs in the LacZ gene of *E-coli* (Watanabe et al., 1993).

The fascinating thing is that sometimes the HA itself as eaten is **metabolically changed by the liver (hepatic microsomes) into active mutagens.** Some research showed that the human liver is more efficient than rat or monkey liver micosomes at metabolizing HA into mutagens (Davis et al., 1993: Brooks et al., 1994). This has intriguing evolutionary implications. When did our human species (the only one that proved viable) actually start to eat cooked food and why has the liver not adapted to it yet.

Patients are surprised when I tell them that the human body needs to be fed mainly raw fat and protein to thrive; no ingested complex carbohydrates are necessary. Cooked carbohydrates (especially complex carbohydrates eaten as grains after baking or frying) offer no extra benefit to the body and result in excess accumula-tion of A.G.E.s (advanced glycation end-products). Since the early 1900's (with studies by Maillard and later Amadori), A.G.E.s have been known through Western medical research to lead to all sorts of common health problems and accelerated aging (Scmidt et al. 1993). More recently (2002) other cancer causing chemicals called acrylamides have been shown to be formed when certain food are heated as in frying or baking. Nature (May 22, 2001) also released similar studies linking the amino acid asparagine when heated in the presence of glucose to acrylamide formation. Particularly high in this carcinogen were potato chips, French fries, baked goods like crackers and pastries, cereals and coffee powder.

As most enzymes are well known to be bent/destroyed at around 117 degrees Fahrenheit, all cooked foods including vegetables can not be digested and assimilated easily. The body does make 1300 enzymes but this requires a shifting of energy from other body parts. Eventually, this attempt to compensate for eating toxic cooked foods results in a systemic degradation commonly seen as a swollen pancreas producing impotent insulin, tired liver and all this implies such as the high incidence of adult onset diabetes and diabetic-like symptoms, digestive problems, heart irregularities etc... .

Some individuals seem to be more susceptible at a physical level, due to the excess quantities of cooked foods they have eaten, to various contaminations through non-organic meat. Secondarily, much of the meat has been contaminated with excessive pesticides. The big problem then becomes when, through pesticides like glyphosate contaminate grain and its ability to rapidly ferment, various chemicals interact within the body of the animal. In an attempt to clean these out, various substances naturally can be produced. These substances may include prions (unique proteins found in most animals including fish but are somehow different when involved in BSE and the human variant Creutzfeldt-Jakob "mad cow" disease (Riviera et al., 1993) and bacteria, which may not be the direct cause of illness but are present during the cleaning out process. When the animal is killed during this cleaning out process, the dangerous cleaning agents are available for ingestion by consumers and sometimes illness will result. Cleaning out of some of these chemicals like tricyclines, chlorofluorocarbons, and other materials that have also broken down through sequence is needed by the body. These toxins are especially a problem when old residues of DDT are present as are persisting in the environment even from the use in the 50's and 60's. These residues are particularly troublesome because their breakdown process is slow, yet, interaction with other substances, in particular, those applied at times to grain, are then interactive.

There was another report released in the January 2004 issue of Science reinforcing what most dietary conscious people have known for years i.e., farmed salmon (actually all farmed fish by nature of their feed) are so toxic that the government is recommending only one helping per month. Toxins and carcinogens reported in Science were polychlorinated biphenyls, dioxins, toxaphene, dieldrin, hexachlorabenzene, lindane, heptachlor epoxide, cis-nonachlor, transnonachlor, gamma-chlordane, alpha-chlordane, Mirex, endrin and DDT. One may want to do more than just say grace before a chemical cocktail like that. Of course, in reality all cooked meals are toxic.

The toxic mercurial levels in dolphins is especially high and Japanese often eat it not knowing how toxic the dolphin meat is (aside from the brutal sickening massacres of the dolphins). When Japanese discover this brutality and toxicity they also will stop eating it. It is so sad to see them buying dolphin in the markets with no warning levels of the mercurial levels which are hundreds of times over the government determined "safe" level.

The much advertised fish-pills do contain omega-3 fatty acids (essentials being DHA, EPA, and ALA) but so do many other whole foods (of course oxidation during the fish oil pill process is a huge concern). These omega 3 fatty acids are in fish only because the fish eat algae which make EPA and DHA. The fish do not synthesis these essential acids. Humans can make both DHA and DPA fatty acids from ALA. Although one hears much about omega-3-acids, omega -6, (and many other fatty acids) are also important and in nature, most fat containing food has a mix of different types of fatty acids. Both omega-3 and omega-6 are also inflammatory by nature (moreso omega-6s as of now) in that they compete for ALA's and lead to eicosanoid production. Eicosanoids are a huge varied group of "local hormones" called eicosanoids eg., prostaglandins, prostacyclines, thromboxanes, leukotrienes, and epoxyeicosatrienoic acids. Eicosanoids are many and varied in purpose and are involved in multiple body systems. They are being studied from many different angles. They have various roles in inflammation, fever, regulation of blood pressure, blood clotting, immune system modulation, control of reproductive processes and tissue growth, and regulation of the sleep/wake cycle (Funk, 2001). Omega-3 and 6s compete for ALA's. Therefore, the ratio of 3s to 6s may be significant.

This is a complex matter, but one must see that there is much more to it than a single organism as there are many levels of contamination associated with the meat that transfers many of these toxins; hence, the importance of organic/natural meat in raw food and aged-meat diets. Only a raw food diet with an adequate number of bacteria strains, raw fats, raw proteins, raw vegetables and some fruits can detoxify the body from the heavy metals, petrochemicals, cooked food toxins and radiation that people inherit first from their parents' genes and then reinforce and compound with an unnatural i.e. cooked diet. Amazingly, one can actually detoxify over time with diet changes; a blessing for those who can see the value and life potential advantages.

The value of raw fats can not be overemphasized. When people understand that every cell in their body, especially the nerves and therefore the brain are high in various lipids/fats, they will more see the need for raw fats, especially the saturated animal fats, in the diet instead of pharmaceuticals which do nothing to build up the nervous system. The body gets about twice as much energy (ATP) from a fat than a carbohydrate or a protein. Heavy metals and some neurotoxins are well known to be fat soluble and thus a scientific natural way to detoxify the body. Avocado, raw butter, cream, raw meat fats and oils are all that most need to start feeling better through an enhanced nervous system, balanced hor-mones, and healthier body. Cooked fats, especially heated polyunsaturated vegetable oils, produce toxins like lipid oxides, acrolein, nitrosamines, hydrocarbons and benzopyrenesa, which are well-known carcinogens (Kabara, 1978).

The media superficially spouts-out the same erroneous health warnings about the dangers of a high cholesterol-fat diet. There is no clear evidence that a high cholesterol or a high fat diet, per se, is not healthful. The often quoted "Framingham Heart Study" clearly did not show any direct relationship between high cholesterol and heart problems. After 40 years, the director of the study said, "In Framingham, MA., those who ate the most saturated fat and cholesterol, weighed the least, were the most physically active, and showed low serum cholesterol" (Archives of Internal Medicine, July 1992, 152:7:1371-1372). The "Framingham Heart Study" did suggest a correlation between a high carbohydrate diet and blood circulation problems. The study showed that weight gain and cholesterol levels had an inverse correlation with fat and cholesterol intake in the diet (Hubert H. et al., 1983). Studies I read while trying to show the benefits of various cholesterol lowering drugs, also include the increased health risks for those who care to read such reports.)

Raw fat are healing and energizing while cooked fats, especially heated vegetable fats, are rancid, mutagenic, or carcinogenic. Plaques in the body are about 50% polyunsaturated vegetable fat products. **The amount of animal fats and cholesterol has decreased in the diet of USA citizens by 20% over the past 50 years and butter consumption has decreased by 75%. Dietary vegetable oils in the form of margarine, shortening, and refined oils have increased by about 400% in the same time period.** Sugar and processed foods have increased by 60%. These numbers (and food research) indicate that saturated animal fats are not the problem but the cure (Enig, 1995).

Saturated fats (including fatty acids like palmitic, butyric, lauric and stearic acids found in animal fats and tropical oils like coconut and palm oil) are called saturated because most or all the available carbon bonds are occupied by a hydrogen atom. This creates stability and means that they do not easily turn rancid. Saturated 18-carbon stearic acid and 16-carbon palmitic acid are the preferred foods for the heart.

The lungs depend on a special lung surfactant phospholipid called dipalmitoyl-phosphatidylcholine which has two saturated fatty acid palmitic acid molecules attached to it; the lung function is dependent on saturated fatty acids. (Bourbon, J.1991). The kidneys rely on saturated fatty acids like myristic, palmitic and stearic acids (Busconi et al. 1997). Fifty percent of animal cell membranes are composed of saturated fats). The body will take fats you eat and place some components into your cell walls. Raw fats lead to healthy cells, and cooked fats lead to toxic cells and lack of biologi-cal functioning. Monosaturated fats (including oleic acid found in nut oils, avocados, and olive oil) lack two hydrogen atoms, but are still relatively stable. Polyunsaturated fats lack four or more hydrogen atoms and are highly reactive and easily turn rancid (oxidize) when heated. Heated polyunsaturated oils are a major cause of toxicity, DNA damage, plaques, and disease in modern diets.

In nature, fats and oils, whether vegetable based or animal based, are some combination of saturated, monounsaturated and polyunsaturated fatty acids. In general, animal fats as in butter, meat and organs are about half saturated fat. Vegetable oils from the tropics are highly saturated. For example, coconut oil is 95 % saturated. Colder climate vegetable oils are mostly polyunsaturated.

In summary, most raw fats and oils are cleansing, energizing and life-enhancing. Cooked fats are carcinogenic, mutagenic and undermine one's biological process which limits one's manifestation of joy and spirituality in life.

Such dietary basic factual knowledge passed on to one's child will also help balance the parent's karma. As stated before, each new generation receives many new genetic mutations passed onto children through the parents' DNA. These mutations can sometimes predispose one to easier activation of various illnesses. Heavy metal toxicity will become known as the root cause of so many illnesses, but as this toxicity is a new post-World War II problem, people must be educated with basic information such as the source of heavy metals. Heavy metals can be molecularly similar to other healthful minerals in the body which causes problems such as when the body takes lead, mistaking it molecularly for calcium, and deposits it in the bone. Sources of contamination are many corporations involved in agricultural, pharmaceutical and insurance work as well as many companies dumping toxic waste into the Earth.

The aluminum and barium added to plane fuel to reduce global warming is also a major health threat worthy of note as these contaminants are in the air and then the ground, soil, plants, animals and finally us. Many studies (e.g., Anway et al. in Science Vol. 308 No.5727) show that environmental toxins, tiny particulate matter (from pollutants) and irradiation can cause systemic inflammatory response and decreased fertility for generations (from F1 to F4).

An incredible pharmacologically researched body of **herbology** has traditionally offered patients much in the way of help, but today there is a well-known problem with heavy metal contamination, which comes naturally, as the plants absorb these toxic metals from the soil and poor processing in Chinese herbs. Nickel, mercury, cadmium, lead etc..., are found in many foods as well as herbs. Many herbs need to be cured or cooked to detoxify them for humans. Alkaloid toxicity has been documented when the curing process was not done properly to hydrolyze toxic aconitine. Even the honey containing the pollen from the *Aconitum spp* plant was blamed for numerous hospital admissions in Japan in 1992. Another cited incident was when a Chinese weight loss preparation caused kidney toxicity as it included the nephrotoxin aristolochic acid from *Aristolochia*, instead of the intended proper alkaloid tetrandrine from the *Stephania;* the two plant names in a Chinese language are similar and the toxin was erroneously added. Finding pure herb sources, as many herb companies are now doing, is an alternative. However, raw foods and less dense foods are, in terms of a longer life for the patient, a greater benefit at many levels for the kidneys and other filtering devices in the body than traditional herbal therapies. I also object to using animal body parts in "herbal" preparations if the animal must be killed just to obtain the parts. I do not doubt the effectiveness of many animal parts in healing.

It is well known in the scientific community that animal testing is of very limited usefulness in human health. In the near future scientists will band together and refuse to use test animals in research.

I have seen incredible healing episodes due to raw food diet implementation over the past few years that would have never been achieved, I believe, without raw foods (including meat) and high bacterial foods. The human body cannot adequately excrete heavy metals and toxic (cooked) food byproducts. I feel that two kidneys are not enough today (we now know nephrons die). Actually, I rarely recommend any conventional supplements and always explain to the patient the toxicity of each supplement as well as the advantage of using it.

The ideal solution is to detoxify ones musculature, organs, glands (and even ones mitochondrial DNA and nucleic DNA) before having children, but this takes years and understandably few are prudent enough to do this. A pill is now marketed for mitochondria DNA repair which includes the well-known and researched alpha-lipoic acid and acetyl L-carnitine. Such nutrients taken as pills are not natural and are chemically inexact copies of the natural chemical (as an example, R-isomer of alpha-lipoic acid is synthesized naturally while S-isomer is not and the two are mixed in pill forms with degraded results. Both these rejuvenating nutrients are found in the highest quantities and potency in raw meats (L-carnitine) and raw organs like heart, kidney and liver (alpha-lipoic acid). Vegetables have a little alpha-lipoic acid and lesser amounts of L-carnitine are in raw milk. These nutrients have been proven to help transport/ chaperone fatty acids into the mitochondria and catalyze reactions for energy and DNA repair (among other functions). **In 2019 low deuterium water became available in the USA and could heal billions.**

Another idea is to detoxify the child as an infant through certain organic/natural raw foods. Babies do wonderfully if raised from day one on raw milk and raw vegetable juice with a little raw honey. Many mothers have take too toxic a diet including cooked foods, medicines and other drugs to advise using their own breast milk. Toxins have long been measurable in women's' breast milk. Raw egg, avocado and banana can be added later to complete the first year of life diet. Of course, no commercially available USA baby formulas or complex carbohydrates are ever recommended (a recent study I read praised baby formula manufacturers in England for having **reduced** the level of toxic dioxins in the formulas dur-ing the 1990s).

Organic Raw meats and high aerobic bacteria diets create a lot of fear and confusion in modern society as people react to erroneous fear-based news stories and do little or no research themselves. I keep raw food at the clinic to feed people so they see how easy and natural it is. (I use natural chocolate syrup in the raw goat milk for people who have issues with the dairy smell or taste). Eating a bit of raw meat, or juicing some vegetables in a blender or draining a coconut together in the clinic often is all people need to start them on a path of healing that would not have happened if someone had not actually done it with them the first time. It breaks a big mental barrier and allows one to access new higher energies that can only be provided when one breaks old patterns and consciously does something different to help themselves. Mental flexibility is essential for growth at all ages and this willingness to change and grow creates many new energetic possibilities that would come either later in life or not at all.

I have advised many adults to eat natural or organic raw meat and not one has ever gotten anything but stronger. Of course, some parents do not want their child to eat meat and that is fine. Raw meat just facilitates and quickens the healing process physically. Also more and more children will reject meat cooked or raw as toddlers. This also is natural for many children and must be respected. Other sources of raw protein from dairy and eggs become more important. Soy milk appears to be the most damaging to children, especially females. Unfortunately, the majority of people willing to do this is already quite ill and does so more out of a sense of desperation than courage or love for themselves or their children. In my experience, the vegetarian diets are just too slow and lack the energizing effects of raw meat inclusion. Most vegetable based food is not organic and thus will contain toxic herbicides, pesticides, and heating them produces toxic resins. Almost all of the non-vegetable food poisoning cases I have read about in and out of the news in the States over the years have been cases of poisoning through canned, cooked and non-organic foods. Many local holistic supermarkets have raw food classes, and there are books and people all over the country following such a "paleo" diet (not to mention millenia of native peoples and carnivorous animals).

As I have written before, getting people to switch to a raw food diet including raw and aged-meat is a unique challenge since the predominant wisdom, the "consensus reality," exerts itself through an emotional tie. Thus, the individual will revert to his or her own feelings which are completely out of proportion to the action involved relating to a few bacteria. It is as if all the fear, all the energies associated with many of the activities of a fear-oriented media have made many feel impotent and afraid. There are so many ways in which the illusions of life itself have been so deeply associated with bacteria at the level of psychology; it is necessary to help them identify their fears and to look at them consciously.

Understanding this principal leads one to a poignant observation: the utilization of chemicals antibiotics and so on, in an attempt to kill bacteria can be understood as bacterial genocide. Bac-teria are an important race and a wise one that coexist with people but have fallen out-of-favor in the popular consensus reality at the current time. However, they exist anyway. Bacteria are already in, on and throughout our bodies and it is simply a matter of find-ing ways to welcome them appropriately. As there are many times more microbes in a human body than there are human cells, and bacterial DNA sequences are in human nucleic DNA, one should ponder on the significance of the implications of this fact when asking what it is to be human. I start most patients on probiotic bacteria pills, which have been around for a long time and one brand now contain up to 35 strains (out of an ever changing estimated 1000s of species in the intestines. There are also hundreds of viruses and fungi in feces specimens). Pills are an easy "non-smelly" way to begin to rebuild the relationship between bacteria and people's consciousness. Eventually, one will need to cultivate by oneself more strains which are not sold and many we cant even grow in a lab. **Eating a tiny fingertip of good organic dirt is still the best way to get enough bacteria into the intestines.**

Major centers all over the country are now testing the healing power of bacteria and viruses for all sorts of healing. Many universities have been using viruses and bacteria to dissolve cancerous tumors and this news is readily available on the internet and in the medical journals. I have witnessed a large cancerous tumour on a mouse be dissolved by a bacterial injection. Some universities that are researching the healing capacities of viruses are Stanford (using the common cold virus), Harvard (using a herpes virus) and Mayo (using a measles virus).

Expensive future expensive therapies can be obviated if people naturally allow themselves and their children to catch various bacteria and viruses while on a raw diet to allow for natural safe cleansing. (It is safer to experience healing viruses and bacteria when the body is on a raw food diet, otherwise the cleaning action can potentially continue too long and in too harsh a manner for the body to withstand).

Again, it must be remembered that if the underlying issues are of fear, it does little good to spend one's time trying to address issues with relationship to science. However, when trying to change someone's underlying reaction to some stimuli in the physical, it must be understood that these reactions are often out of the individual's conscious control.

Fortunately around 2019 low deuterium water became available in the USA and I think that this will heal many human illnesses. Earth water now has about 150ppm deuterium and this is not healthful. Research and now many patients have shown that lowering one's Deuterium level (I measure through saliva) to below 130ppm allow the mitochondria in every cell to function well and this heals a lot . (Now in 2019 prices vary for various ppm water eg., 250US$ for five gallons of 25ppm water, dilute it with regular water to 100ppm and drink 2-3 liters a day and after 4 months you need much less judging from patients' saliva tests. I test the water I buy to verify it is at the labeled ppm! I also test all my patients saliva before and after after three months to verify their level is down to 100-130ppm. As for food, only fat is low in deuterium (80-100) so a high raw fat diet like in the Primal diet is perfect. Raw Organic Coconut Cream and Dairy Cream are the favorite high fat foods by far, followed by Raw Organic Bacon.)

Of the 1000s of bacterial strains we believe humans need to be healthy and happy, many produce the hormones/neurotransmitters we all crave to be healthy and happy i.e., dopamine, serotonin and GABA. Bacteria will be important in the future of healing and depression. I believe, from personal experience, that only ORGANIC SOIL will provide enough bacteria to heal humans. A fingertip-worth of organic soil is plenty.

The 90 minute lymph detox bath WITH coconut cream and pineapple is one of the best scientific ways to heal. Human fat melts at 104.5 farenheit in about 45 minutes. The fat stores many toxins like pthalates and as the fat melts many toxins can leave the body over the next 45 minutes. Also, as you monitor your body temperature you will see the water induces a fever which heats the blood and allows for some brain detox as all fevers do. Increased antigen presentation also happens. Many listen to music, meditate, watch tv etc but as long as u get it done. Great to have the inert gas device in the area as well as any scalar wave-sound frequency device also. The fever can last a while or come and go after the bath and the bath is draining for many people for 24 hours but you do adapt a bit after a few baths and by the 30th to 40th bath huge changes can be scene- especially with lymphoma. You will need to drink a few bottles (4-8) of water while in the bath and more afterward. It is a life changer and the one key part to healing that many never do till they are terminal. **The organic raw diet is not enough to heal many things without the baths.** Various types of rejuvenation likewise do not seem to be possible without the baths.

A good way to start the organic raw diet is to do what's easier. For most , that means veggie juicing, raw milk, and less cooked food each day. Just those 2 things can bring good changes and start to realign one's consciousness to the reality that highly heated food is often carcinogenic and living in a state of unconscious starvation is not a way to be healthy and evolve.

As one start to feel better or different they often want to feel even better. Since raw animal fats increase some hormonal production, natural or organic raw butter or cream usually increases the labido and for men the prostate fluid production. If one really wants to start helping the musculature and organs then raw organic meat will be best. Raw organic red meat like ground beef or bacon are easiest for many and raw bacon actually tastes good and has always been a favorite with raw food people. One can add spices or saute it but I just eat it plain. Even one bite a day is enough to start changing energetic pathways. Likewise raw organic white meat is fowl so chicken and turkey are common. Turkey tastes fine as is but chicken is preferred by most soaked in lemon juice and spice like ginger. The lemon juice makes chicken taste good and the texture also softens.

Just experimenting with some of these foods can be a life changer and open up your possibilities in life. One's soul often waits a lifetime for you to show some self love and respect by eating non-toxic food. Eating cancer-causing food daily reflects self-loathing that only degrades one's vitality and limits one's consciousness to the illusionary reality that surrounds us. Eating cooked is part of the repetitive mass trap to keep humans enslaved in their 3d limited malnourished " life."

I always thank the animal that I am eating and I know one day I will become healthy enough and evolved enough to not need meat. I was taught by my Kagyu teachers that animals have decided on a group soul level, in a last desperate attempt, to offer themselves up to humans hoping that humans will acquire some of the animal understanding and and instincts and realign with nature so that humans stop destroying Mother Earth. This offering also limits humans' karmic debt taken on by eating animals.

DIETARY BASICS

Carcinogens and mutagens are produced by highly heating food-meat, fat, grains etc (see intro and pg 82)

Enzymes are ruined my very low heat(average 115F)

Resins in cooked vegetables are toxic

The Brain is 60% dry weight fat and half of that is animal fat

Pesticides and herbicides are on grains, fruits and vegetables
(90% of breads, cereals, and alcohol contain glyphosate)

Microbes are designed to clean human bodies of toxins

Bacteria produce happy chemicals like Serotonin & Dopamine

Human DNA includes a lot of viral, bacterial and parasitical DNA

Therefore eating organic raw: meat, dairy, fruits,veggies, fats and ingesting 1000s of bacterial strains will produce a happy healthy human. The brain especially needs a lot of animal fat to allow for ideal function and happy mental health neurotransmitters.

REFERENCES

Brooks RA et al. PhIP is a potent carcinogen in mouse small
intestine. *Cancer Res* 54:1165-1171 1994

Bourbon, Jacques. Lung Surfactant: biochemical, functional and
clinical concepts. CRC Press 1991

Busconi et al., *Biochem J* 1997:327

Davis C. et al. Studies of mutagenic activation of HAs by
monkey, rat and human microsomes. *Cancer Let.*73:95 1993

Funk, Colin. "Prostaglandins and Leukotrienes: Advances in in
Eicosanoid Biology." *Science* 294 11-30-2001 (5548): 1871–1875

Grote, D. et al. Live attenuated measles virus induces

regression of human lymphoma xenografts in immunode
ficient

mice. *Blood* 97: 3746-3754 (2001)

Kabara, J, The Pharmaceutical Effects of Lipids, 1978 1-14
The Lancet, 1998, 352:688-91

Knize MG. et al. Analysis of cooked meats for heterocyclic
aromatic amine carcinogens,. *Mutat Res.* 376:129-34 1997

Rivera-Milla E. et al. An evolutionary basis for scrapie
disease; identification of a fish prion mRNA Trends in
Genetics, 19: 72-75, (2003).

Schmidt et al, Stern Cellular receptors for advanced glycation
end products; implications for induction for oxidant stress and
cellular dysfunction in the pathogenesis of vascular lesions
Arteriosclerosis and Thrombosis, 1994, Vol.14 (10):1521-8
J Nephrology 2001; 13 (suppl. 3) (S83-S88)

Wakabashi K, Ushiyama H. et al. Exposure to heterocyclic
amines *Environ Health Perspective*, 99:129-134 1993 Wakabashi
K. et al. Food-Derived mutagens and carcinogens

carcinogens, *Cancer Res*, 52(7 Suppl): 2092-2098 1992

Watanabe M. et al. Analysis of mutational specificity by
    HA in lac z gene of E. coli. Cancer 14:149-153 1993

White, A. Pesticides in Food Journal of Environmental
    Pathology, *Toxicology and Oncology* 13:163-168. 1986

Yuan B. et al. Mutation and repair induced by carcinogen
    PhIP in Chinese hamster ovarian cells. *Chem Res
    Toxicology* 7:209-218 1994

American Society for Microbiology General Meeting May
2001 Florida. *Nature* News Science MacMillan Ltd. 2001
"FDA Launches Plan to Reduce Acrylamides in Foods."

Reuters Health press release 9-30-02

The Development of Human Consciousness through the Spiritual Energy of Organs

Chinese medical/philosophical theory proposes that there are twelve main organs in the body, and these twelve are grouped into six pairs of one yin organ (heart, liver, pericardium, spleen/pancreas, lungs and kidneys) and one yang organ (small intestine, gall bladder, triple warmer, stomach, large intestines and bladder). The six groupings are:

heart/small intestine ,	kidney/bladder
pericardium/triple-warmer, lungs/large intestine	liver/gallbladder sspleen/stomach

---

There is an intimate energetic relationship between these organs and they help balance each other biochemically. The 12 acupuncture meridians reflect not just organ function but also various endocrine gland functions. This is not taught in any USA schooling but more intuitive practitioners have evolved into this glandular understanding. The advantages and insights of working in a busy Asian clinics with senior clinicians seeing 50 patients a day is why all students in the USA should do so for years but few actually do. Most Western clinicians I have met lack this large patient body experience and may never reach the level of an experienced clinician. For most there is no substitute for clinical experience with senior clinicians and that generally wont be found in the USA so it is up to the serious prudent student to go to Asia AFTER preparing and planning how to do so. Some Americans go for a week or a month but that is just a crude intro. It takes years. One has to live within the Asian community and have studied the local language and whichever martial art is in that area before going to Asia to really be welcomed into the Asian community and be taught the most important guarded clinical or temple or doujou teachings.

Clinically one often sees how an imbalance in one of the paired organs affects its yin/yang counterpart as in the constipated asthmatic (large intestine/lung) or the enzymatic deficient person with digestive problems (spleen/pancreas stomach) or the burning urination of certain kidney imbalances (bladder/kidney). Now there are even deeper less understood relationships between these organs and some of these relate to emotional and spiritual development of the organ and the person. These are little talked about and almost never taught, as usually they must be intuited clinically. Remember that much wisdom has never been translated or even written. Much of Oriental medical schooling is based on a few texts which, although wonderful, are from comprehensive and sufficient texts for those seeking deeper answers.

The issue of the relationship between an organ and a human's development goes beyond mere health, as the very process of human evolution is determined in part by how people, as enlightened humans, consciously choose to understand, develop and manifest the spiritual energies inherent in each organ. Many people have done this unconsciously, but the conscious connection usually begins with a medical diagnosis because an organ is deficient and the person is "sick." A person then starts to study and learn the functions of the organ. Though these functions would normally be available on a primarily medical or anatomical level, they will remind the individual very much of the similar issues in their life. Unfortunately, most people do not make this connection and miss the great healing path made available to them by a medical imbalance. I usually try to talk with patients about how their symptoms relate to their stagnation in some area of life e.g. intestinal imbalances often physically relate to how the body is having problems excreting food matter that the body cannot utilize at that stage.

Emotionally/psychologically intestinal imbalances often relate to how an individual is having difficulty letting go of old ideas/emotions (post-digested foodstuff) etc...to make room for new ones (new nutrients).

How one reacts to the need for changing one's ideas will determine whether one experiences diarrhea or constipation etc....
This relationship can be seen with every organ and gland and its related emotional/psychological block. Many patients are very interested in this relationship and start working on their own healing immediately. However, these layers of healing and blockages can get frustrating as one works through emotional/psychological stagnation to allow for new realizations, so one must be patient. Just knowing the impaired organ's function and its emotional connection is a major step but by no means the end to a physical problem. Many people will recognize the truth when given correct information about their body, even if it is just a subtle inkling.

The important symbiotic role of bacteria and other microorganisms in human evolution must be considered. Anti-biotics can be seen as suicidal/genocidal in nature and ingesting high bacteria foods as reflective of self-love. When the meaning of this statement is really understood, consciousness augments and healing is expedited.

However, the main problem is that most people are unable to recognize the inherent symbolic significance of the organs and the physical body and the person, personality, awareness etc....
These basic symbolic connections are difficult for most people to understand and accept because they have to a large extent rejected the underlying significance. Sometimes it is the significance of the

animal body, sometimes it is the significance of that issue in their life — they are moving into a position of denial. Denial of various important issues can be a useful path towards awareness but such a path begins with ignorance, pushing away and only then one recognizes that a mistake has been made and then learning can occur.

It does make sense to consciously work with the energies by consciously "running" energy and colors through the meridians. Many patients enjoy this visualization and find it easy to do as it gives them a controllable and eventually kinesthetic understanding of energy. The meridians are mostly linear and easy to remember by looking at acupuncture meridian pictures and models (see acupuncture chart in appendix). People usually start at the lowest number point on any meridian and imagine some color or sensation moving through the meridian in Western numerical order to the "couple" point which is a special acupuncture points where energy on one organ's pathway/meridian naturally connects to the next organ's meridian.

As an example, one could start with Lung meridian point number one on the chest and imagine energy flowing down the arm (the lung pathway) to the thumb area where it joins with the point that connects it to the large intestine pathway. The point of this simple practice is to tune-up the physical body by learning to work with the more subtle energies. It is an effective exercise as one can actually feel something if one keeps practicing.

It is most difficult when someone is working against some underlying issue, some habit pattern, something that they have denied at an emotional level or some level that relates more to higher aspects of their lives than simply the physical. The result of this struggle can be a sort of reshuffling of many priorities and a deeper acceptance of the animal-self; the very basic primitive aspects which are most powerful and at the same time least understood by a majority of people with whom I have worked with regard to the organs, the glands and the physical components. Martial art training and raw foods (especially natural/organic raw meats and organs) are a great advantage in developing this connection. (Please see section on martial art training.)

This type of thinking reflects very clearly in the brain, and a greater understanding of the brain will eventually yield all information as a true symbolic connection. The brain itself relates to consciousness but consciousness has many different forms. It is not just the form of the awareness that people are most familiar with i.e., the forms of consciousness that include different types of learning and different intelligences as have been studied by so many. What eventually emerges is a powerful understanding of emotional consciousness and emotional intelligence. The result of this is an awareness that takes one back to the physical as there will be an emotional connection that will usually be felt physically and, therefore, into the associated organs and glands.

The point is to allow consciousness itself to develop in several different ways as if to involve emotional consciousness, animal consciousness, territorial awareness, the interaction of the various aspects in life leading at the deeper level to the understanding and awareness that comes from the organs themselves, as if recognizing their innate intelligence and then later the glands (and this inevitably leads to the chakras and miasms and their connections to the higher aspects).

Another subtle energetic problem I see with many sensitive people is that as they attune to "global consciousness" (initially subconsciously as we all do) there is an increased sense of anxiety and fear that the person cannot explain. This reception of global worries can cause much consternation and energy loss until one learns what is happening and how to deal with it. **As** the world vortexes speed up and according to modern physics, time actually moves faster as the universe expands more rapidly (1), naturally there can be a lot of stress as people sense the foreboding energies that surround us — as humans' fear and confusion is transmitted through the ethers. It is easy to understand such anxiety as people are imbued with scare tactics and misinformation about terrorism, disease, economics and scarcity on a daily basis.

For many who are inherently ultra-sensitive or psychic, this attunement to global-consciousness is felt as a sense that is akin to a type of "homesickness" or longing. This feeling is the need for the connection to the larger family i.e., humanity as a connected living unit. All of the powerful issues that many are concerned with in the world become difficult for such people to properly balance. This moves naturally in various sequences. Moving into times when, as a global people are struggling, so also will an individual struggle.

Working this out is always difficult when one attempts to do this by logical means. It is just too big for any single human consciousness. Processes of meditation, inner attunement and especially deep inner quiet, mind chatter stilling completely, become so important. These beautiful processes allow one to merge with the global consciousness and whatever facet of it is necessary. These are energies of innate consciousness, essence of the universe that is manifested in different ways to different people. However, these energies cannot be received by thinking or even feeling. Moving to such a special place of quiet can be easy once one has regularly established the methodology but, as many have sensed, the "global-consciousness" is shifting with regards to these modalities. What a fun challenging time in which to be living!

In the brain is the source of the manifestation of every aspect of the body. It is the source of expression for the growing consciousness that shapes and forms everything. Spirit manifests through the brain in the creation of thought and ideas and many other energies that shape our physicality. **That is to say that the source of human intelligence is not local. It is as though the brain were a transformer of incoming energies that over evolution have shaped it physically in order to adapt human consciousness.**

The acupuncture and Indian meridians/nadis reflect the action of distribution of energy absolutely necessary for the health of the physical body. This is an automatic function. When one has spiritual breakthrough, the energy will naturally be transferred. Spiritual breakthrough for most individuals is exceptionally difficult if one is seeking to understand two different aspects of consciousness or awareness — three aspects would be nearly impossible. This difficulty is reflected in individuals' tremendous difficulty with a 100% focused concentration on any single idea or single thought. When one is able to crystallize thought to the point that one can become more consciously aware of this energy, it is much easier for the individual to properly integrate it and work with it. Yet, it is this one-pointed concentration, this deeper immersion that is so necessary for deeper states of enlightenment or understanding. As a result, some individuals who focus only on the technique of one-pointed concentration without any direct attunement towards spiritual awareness, understanding bigger principals, working with spirit energy, meditation etc..., achieve states of enlightenment and understanding simply because they have mastered one-pointed focus. The nature of spiritual breakthrough under most circumstances is a letting go, not an adding to.

The spiritual energy, the aspect of Spirit, is assumed to permeate all manifestation. Many blocks to this are present within consciousness. There are many reasons why the individual dwells upon the past or the future; it is in vain, as it draws one's attention away from the present where all of the joy, all of the energy, all of the intuition and all of the aspects of existence are. Yet, one continues to do so out of habit because even knowing the difficulties, they persist. By example, you see how the block to the present is so available simply by habit patterns of attention on the future or the past. One must through meditation learn how to access the energy that is always present by one-pointed focus on the present. Hence, the paradox that the spiritual energy, which is present everywhere, is best received by a singular focus because this simply draws away the blocking energies.

Simplification is best for most people nowadays. However, as I have seen with so many patients, wherever there can be this attunement to emptiness there is always tremendous benefit to their consciousness because as the body is given any of the raw materials available — be it energy through meditation, raw foods or sufficient strains of bacteria — it seems to be able to construct various bridges between right and left brain, manifest new energetic patterns and create long lasting positive change!

As an example of this emotional/physical component, I will explain some aspects of the pairing of the
heart and the small intestine in Oriental theory. I believe
that the understanding of this special pairing is essential
for human development now more than ever. This pairing is the least understood and discussed at all levels of
education.

In certain philosophical systems, the heart/small intestine
pairing has to do with the end of a cycle and the beginning of a
new one. In other systems it has to do with the awareness of the in
and out with regard to the entire consciousness. That is, the small
intestine relating to the issues of absorbability, receiving and integration; the heart relating to the capacity of the creation of love and
the ability to release it. Such in and out are indeed wide extremes,
yet, the heart is not intrinsically yang nor is the small intestine intrinsically yin, it serves both functions as they both do and in this
way a deeper balance usually emerges.

However, as meridians this pairing is concerned with energy
flow and the ability of the flow to shift. The most important aspect
relates to the functional quality as impressed upon one or the other
organ. That is, the heart is missing some of the qualities associated
with absorption and small intestine, and the small intestine missing
some of the qualities of love relating to the heart so in that sense
they are perfect matches.

As for the heart's physiological manifestation of lacking small
intestine absorptive qualities, there is often difficulty with proper
functioning. Typical responses are heart murmur, arrhythmia, in-
ability for the heart to come to full growth being too small or in

some cases too large, an imbalance between the heart and other components of the body. Secondarily, the entire circulatory system and eventually the heart itself can over-respond to insulin. This over-response can lead to many difficulties and eventually to heart attack itself where rapid fibrillation causes muscle degeneration. In addition, there can be susceptibility within the heart muscle itself to various microorganisms and ways in which this reduces heart functioning, causing breakdown of various walls and again leading to such as arrhythmia heart murmur etc.... The extra meridians are of much use in balancing the heart energy.

As for the small intestine's physiological manifestation of love, it is a way in which self-love and the ability to receive the support from the environment is not properly utilized. Specifically, this involves the materials that are utilized in the physical body trying to penetrate directly into the blood through the duodenum. The way in which the small intestine must work on the final digestive process requires that such be an integrative loving process. Where these energies can happen too quickly or too slowly, there can be some difficulty. In addition, there can be the formation of polyps as referring then to various areas in which love has been rejected, held back, not allowed more consciously and this love specifically relating to the energies from others, their ability to love and assist through their own support, their conscious recognition and their interaction with others. Acid/alkaline imbalances can result in various yeasts in the small intestine as a healing modality but here again an observance of the rejection or resistance to the opportunity to absorb that love. The absorptive quality is always important but it is the individual's ability to more consciously work with absorption; that is, consciously take in the love, consciously work with it as it is provided by others, that will often influence the small intestine. (It took me a long time to understand the real meaning behind my Elders' constant advice that I could love better if I ate better. I would for years nod/bow my head in acknowledgement without adequately understanding their meaning.)

The body reflects nature and this can be seen in fractal geometric formations which were well known in Asian art (centuries before modern mathematicians like Benoit B. Mandelbrot "discovered" fractal geometry in the West). One sees this in many art works—especially Tibetan and Buddhist mandalas. The heartbeat, when graphed out also reflects a fractal formation. Biofeedback and software can be used to entrain people to more healthy brainwave and heart beat patterns. The heart energy can also be influenced in this way, but many times it is an energy that is much more intrinsic relating to the sense of family, of the little child in oneself, the loving self the child self being that which influences. Actions of belief patterns,

Working-out issues in the world and so on as one comes more into adulthood can be more focalized in the small intestine. Hence, you will see more problems developing in later life relating to small intestine issues, whereas some of the heart issues, particularly those associated with birth defect will be noted early in life.

Much of the Chinese process and the use in acupuncture of the treatment of small intestine meridian and organ for spinal and brain imbalances revolve around "Five Element Theory" and the transfer of these energies in other ways. The development of the calcium ion appropriately in the physical body depends on many energies of a subtle nature. Those elements that can be derived from small intestine meridian stimulation appear to best strengthen this capacity for proper absorption and utilization of calcium. In addition, spinal difficulty will often revolve around certain specific issues relating to structure in one's life, a sense of support and being helped and connected to others and assisted through their actions. Small intestinal actions often relate to one's ability to connect to the world. The whole principal of final absorption in this way with the outside world and others will also therefore at the level of the etheric body effect interaction of the spinal formation. Spinal cord itself is to some extent influenced here as well. Although this is more of a nervous system interaction, it does directly relate to the way in which the spinal cord is able to move grow and shift and in this way affect some of the bony structure. In addition, small intestine energy will at times displace various ideas related to issues around which individuals have blocked absorption. These ideas as fixed ideas reduce circulation through many of the energy centers in the back and spine (where the small intestine energy channel runs). These are directly related to the larger concept of a signature or functional aspect — that of the support structure of the back. So, as these ideas or fixed energies are shifted, the energy becomes more flexible, more available and therefore, as a result, more easily transferred in and around the back (again, my Elders' succinct teaching, in broken English, was "bend back-bend thinking")

An area of research in much need of attention is the issue of bacterias' roles in healing the body and the intimate relation to the small intestine bacteria count and depression. There are at present estimates, 1000s of types of beneficial bacteria in our intestines, each having many strains that have been identified. (2) Some are aerobic (needing air) and some are anaerobic (not needing air) and some are lactic acid producing and can be aerobic and anaerobic. These bacteria control much of our health and sense of feeling good. These bacteria directly stimulate endocrine cells in the small intestine to produce chemicals like serotonin (and many others) that make one feel happy. Patients are surprised when I tell them that 90% of serotonin is produced in the gut. These bacteria help control our acid/alkaline balance, which also influences our moods and health. These bacteria balance each other, feed each other, and allow for all sorts of sharing of DNA and polymorphisms (bacteria changing forms). A shortage of bacteria in the gut leads to poor health of body and mind. These bacteria can directly produce dopamine, serotonin etc. Others signal the brain to produce the same.

There are various ways in which an increase of bacterial strains and manifestation of appropriate bacteria in the intestinal tract with fixed periods of depression and long periods of stress will cause a sort of concretization or strengthening of various harming energy vortices in the body. These can often relate to the back to remind an individual that they must have some new sup-port structure, must relate better to other people or find a way of greater flexibility in the structures that they are creating for them-selves. When this deterioration in health goes on too long, there is a cleansing reaction that has the form of various bacteria that lead to various difficulties to experience pain as arthritis. The bacte-ria are attempting to clean out some of the deposited toxic mate-rial and this can often be problematic in the back area. Sometimes these problems will be perceived, before arthritis is diagnosed, as a more typical problem occurring in the joints of the feet or hands as so often seen in the clinic. However, when one has the recognition of the back difficulties, one can sometimes make some early cor-rections and here just talking with the patient can be of assistance. In addition, absorption of one particular mineral, manganese (3), is strongly influenced by the small intestine, as that is where it is absorbed. It is able to allow and govern flow and the metal element itself generally balanced on many levels. Ultimately, this rebalancing of the small intestine to get properly absorbed manganese into the body is an important catalyst at proper formation of bones and nerves, thus, reducing pain and creating a balancing. This is why at times there can be immediate relief of pain with ingestion of high levels of manganese as a cheated mineral. Long term this produces kidney problems because with an excess of this material only a small amount can be absorbed. However, short term it can be very helpful. I have repeatedly found that homeopathic manganese at the 12x potency provides a small amount physically while at the same time encouraging the individual to release stuck issues and to shift their relationships so others can support them and this allows for a dual cleansing.

The brain itself has little interaction with bacteria. There are many ways in which bacteria cannot easily cross the blood brain barrier. It is in the small intestine that many chemicals are produced that are inherent soothing materials: neuropeptides, all kinds of ph (hydrogen potential) balancers, substances that moderate the affects of adrenaline, noradrenalin, blood sugar swings, even production of DMT (a strong hallucigenic) in the pineal.(4) All of these substances have a constant level of interactivity and the way the actions in the small intestine govern these always seem to return to bacteria and the way in which they are able to naturally come to a state of homeostasis and balance with the brain produced chemicals. The brain itself produces chemicals, some moving in ways that are problematic for the small intestine so usually it takes a while before homeostasis is struck. However, in the formation of wide varieties of bacteria one is relying on the innate intelligence of the body to line up properly and work with those materials during the process of transition. Sometimes such a transition process can take years as various psychic imbalances or troublesome psychological conditions gradually balance to the point that the individual no longer needs the extra bacteria. As the brain moves through various changes, it will also either release chemicals itself or cause the other glands, in particular the adrenals, to produce materials that can destroy some of the sensitive bacteria only at a delicate stage in its development in the small intestine. This is why repeated dosing of the small intestine with proper bacteria is necessary. Examples of this adrenal interference are manic depression, bipolar disorder or various forms of depression in which the individual is producing lower levels of adrenalin than are necessary in the body and then swinging to much higher ones.

However, the larger picture is one of genetic incompletion as there are other meridians that exist at a higher energetic level. These are not yet brought into DNA, but we as humans can speed this up a bit by understanding these deeper realities. One can visualize and intuit various components of this occurring in different ways resulting in many additional new meridians instead of the present commonly known and taught twelve meridians.

These new meridians would likely begin with a special energy flow (meridian) relating to the flows of energy corresponding to the heart and small intestine. These newly focused energies would eventually give rise to another extra meridian. These two extra meridians would flow in both directions; that is, one moving up/down in the body, the other moving crossways in the body and interknitting these different capacities. Indeed, as anyone proficient in energy direction will say, this is one of the most difficult of energy flows particularly at the couple points on the extremities where there is a big shift of energy from heart to small intestine. This bridging is a difficult one for many to understand. In fact, it is one of the places where a number of significant difficulties in both the organs will often have its very earliest starting point at the ability to make these shifts. It is for this reason that lingering in massage or attention on the hands and feet in these areas can be helpful in diagnosing imbalances. As the extra meridians start to come in this may ease as people consciously attune to these energies and their spiritual implications.

Physical changes in the body would also be likely as new meridians manifest. These physical changes would have to relate to spiritual integration as the important characteristic to be added but one can think of this also as relating to the "12 plex," as the great importance of this has already been observed for ages as in the Mayan and other mathematical systems. Anyone who has had the honor to treat some of the "enlightened children" in various parts of the world (hopefully with parents initiated enough to understand somewhat the significance of their child's extra meridians) is honored to have had such an encounter. Understanding the relationship of all of this takes one way beyond the mere meridians, but is a way in which it can all make sense as healers meditate and sensitize themselves to these concepts. At a place of unity, of course, all of these distinctions disappear and there is a way then there is a singular flow more as a vortex.

Part Three References

1. Science Journal 2-27-98. The Associated Press announced in 1998 that the discovery of the accelerating galaxies was picked by the editors of 'Science' as the top scientific advance in 1998.

2. Macfarlane, G, and J.H. Cummings. "Probiotics and Pre-biotics: Can Regulating the Activities of Intestinal Bacteria Benefit Health?" British Medical Journal 318 (10 April 1999): 999-1003

3. Komura, J. Sakamoto, M (1992) Effects of Manganese Forms on Biogenic Amines in the Brain and Behavioral Alterations. Environmental Research, 57, 34-44

4. Shukla, G.S. (1976) Effect of Manganese on the levels of DNA and RNA in Cerebrum, Cerebellum and Brain. Acta Pharmacology, 43, 562-564

CASE STUDIES

ALL cases involve the most important basics of various inert gas combinations, raw foods(meat, dairy, veggies, fruit, bacteria and a few can work with viruses), sound frequency therapy via scalar waves and, most recently (2019), the low deuterium water that has become available. These technologies offer the best hope for human evolution and health. The deuterium depleted water(DDW) by itself, will heal so many "DIS-EASES."

Case #1:

An attention/ learning disorder

Nobody realizes that some people expend tremendous energy merely to be normal.

—Albert Camus

This was a case of a seven-year-old boy with a Western medical diagnosis of a type of so-called "A.D.H.D." (attention deficit hyperactive disorder). He could not express himself clearly in typical conversation. His limited elocution was fine but he used abbreviated sentence structure and spoke too quickly when he did speak. The boy was in partial special education classes that do at times provide a somewhat loving atmosphere at best but are not equipped to help in the healing of such children. The boy's mother had decided not to use medication on her son; this was a brave faithful move on the mother's part as there were other children in the family and all the conflicts such a child brings into a family are uniquely challenging. However, a negative response to stimulant medicine (methylphenidate eg., Ritalin and amphetamine eg., Adderall) would have helped rule-out ADHD. Stimulant drugs are very effective at controlling many ADHD symptoms and are often used for differential diagnosis. There is a growing body of empiricism and research supporting the idea that stimulant medicines are leading to a significantly increased number of pediatric cardiac and psychiatric cases. (This resulted in the Food and Drug Administration (FDA) mandate for medication guides to alert patients to potential cardiovascular risks and adverse psychiatric symptoms. Almut Gertrud Winterstein, PhD, from the Department of Pharmaceutical Outcomes and Policy at the College of Pharmacy, and the Department of Epidemiology and Biostatistics at the College of Public Health and Health Professions, University of Florida, Gainesville, and colleagues write in *Pediatrics* (July 2009) that clinical trial data have shown evidence of cardiac adverse effects, including increases in heart rate and blood pressure and case reports of cardiac sudden death, in children exposed to stimulants. In addition, the authors published a recent cohort study of more than 50,000 children with ADHD that showed a 20% increased risk for cardiac ED visits for all stimulants combined.) One must be careful to realize that most people feel better on stimulants (which is why they are sold illegally and parents use their child's medicine) but in ADHD patients these drugs allow for increased attention-spans and concentrated study resulting in increased self-esteem and less psychological scarring.

This patient had wonderful hazel-colored eyes, was handsome, physically skinny (underweight), weak in muscular strength and lacking in coordination upon testing but otherwise not particularly uncoordinated in everyday movements-and he could run well. He slept well and rarely caught colds. No notable medical history in his family. He had no known family hx of rage, suicidal ideation, violence, abuse, ADHD or any psychiatric disorder. He presented as happy and overly playful. He was difficult to engage with poor eye contact. He was generally alert, happy, smiled often and liked animals. Initially, he would not answer questions or ask questions of me. His facial morphology and symmetry were unremarkable. Initially I considered a processing disorder or even some subtle type of pervasive development disorder. Unfortunately, he had not been formally tested to evaluate his general cognitive ability such as information processing and IQ/intelligent quotient (eg. Wechsler Scales/Tests and the Achenbach Child Behavior Check List) which is always valuable information to have as it gives an assigned number we use for comparison for verbal comprehension, perceptual reasoning, memory, and processing. (The Full Scale IQ is derived from ten sub-scores, and is generally considered the most representative estimate of global intellectual function and standard traditional academic education potential. It is important to remember that many tests must be carefully analyzed as academically challenged students can place in the superior range of intellectual ability if, for example, the perceptual reasoning score is high while placing much lower in verbal comprehension and processing speed. In such a case the cognitive potential would be high while the deficit between ability and achievement scores would lean toward a type of learning disability. IQ tests are indicative of academic potential in present day schooling. IQ does not evaluate creativity, artistry, character, personality, likes and dislikes, leadership, motivation, dreams, niceness, sweetness, charm, sense-of-humor, spirituality, wisdom etc…)

The first issue was to gain trust and compatibility between the child and myself. He would often dart from the room, try to put paper on the incense, and excessively repeat certain phrases. Since we could not really converse verbally for many weeks, we communicated in more simple subtle ways. I asked him to look me in the eyes more when we spoke. He did this willingly, and his eye energy was strong— as though he longed to look directly at someone as well as be looked at directly. After just a few treatments, his mom could leave the treatment/play room and we would be fine by ourselves. He held my hand at times and when he went under the seven foot by seven foot pyramid to relax and practice the medita-tion, he would often fall asleep. His mother was surprised that he could sleep in the daytime let alone in a newer environment.

I approached things playfully but at times strictly, as such children tend to be a bit destructive, messy or try to run out of the treatment room suddenly and need some fun restraint with the parent's permission or presence. Physically holding (restraining) them while joking or playing a game is common (fortunately most of our pediatric cases are male). This usually produces laughter as long as trust has been established. Initially we would chant a bit and listen to various sacred music to see what he liked. He preferred Native American flutes.

Initially, his usual reply to most of my questions would be, "I don't know." I interpreted his instant reactive answer as a neuronal (brain circuit) connection that had become fixed due to repetition and had become a set habit pattern. This connection needed to be broken and recircuited mechanically by repetitive practice. I took this as his needing affirmation that he could do many things and that he was not lacking in intelligence even though he knew he was in special classes.

He also began to ask me questions. He had a favorite question he would tend to ask out of habit, which was, "How's your broken finger?" (I have had many broken bones from years of martial art training in Asia and one had healed noticeably bent and this interested him). He wanted to try to fix my pinky finger so he treated me with guided assistance of acupuncture needles and lasers. During each treatment, we repeated many times that he was special. Indeed, in a wonderful way that is hard for others to understand. I would initially ask him, "who's special?" and he would say, "I don't know." Then after a few weeks, he would reply that he was special or his stuffed animal was special. After six weeks he would never say, "I don't know," when asked, "Who's special?" He would continue to mischievously reply that his toys were special knowing that I would pretend to be exasperated (as I would often do when he replied with any old fixated energy words). He had a wonderful gleeful laugh that aided him energetically.

He took quickly to receiving acupuncture needles (as do most children). Upon needle insertion he often replied "Look, I got some energy." Eventually as part of his therapy of increasing his sense of self-empowerment and caring for others he was allowed to put a needle into his stuffed toys (which he would always bring with him to the clinic and needed to have close to him). He showed kindness in needling his stuffed animals and never exhibited any hint of meanness or cruelty. He also enjoyed using and receiving the various cold lasers (again, as do most children).

(In 2003, the FDA approved "cold" low level **lasers** based, in part, on research done to treat carpal tunnel syndrome patients. I have always used lasers for many conditions, and taught my patients to use these simple safe lasers on themselves and their children.

The lasers which were tested and approved were in the 670nm range which the eye perceives as in the red spectrum. Interestingly, this 670nm is the same frequency that 40.00$ pen lasers function at, and are an inexpensive effective option to some of the more expensive 670nm lasers being marketed for medical use (Japanese ITO produces a 120.00$ 670nm inexpensive medical diode laser). I usually prefer the more biologically appropriate inert gas 634.5 lasers, as this frequency has been measured as a cellular frequency emitted during certain biological mechanisms. I have gotten the best results using inexpensive helium-neon inert gas lasers which include 634.5nm.

There are various size **needles** in length and width. In the West, disposable small stainless steel needles are popular and recommended. Japanese laser-tipped stainless steel needles are favored by many practitioners even though, at 10.00$ for a box of 100 individually packaged, they are twice as expensive as Chinese or Korean stainless steel needles. Japanese acupuncture styles often use smaller needles and more subtle needling techniques as well as theoretically complex treatment plans. In some Japanese styles, needles of different alloys such as gold, silver, copper and zinc are used. Needles are sometimes not left in the body (or inserted at all). A tonification and or dispersal technique is used. I often ordered special gold needles for older Asian patients who knew of the tonification properties of a metal like gold. The Chinese styles often use larger needles or more aggressive needling techniques. Reusing the same needles after sterilizing them in an autoclave was done everywhere until the 1990s (and still done in poorer countries) and is quit safe. Many foreigners would bring their own needles.

We later started him on the usual right-left brain coordination exercises with opposite limbs moving in opposite directions simultaneously. This practice is an easy and direct way to connect the right and left brain hemispheres. The corpus callosum in many children isn't developed well and cant conduct messaging between the 2 brain hemispheres (since the brain/nerves are 60% dry weight fat, raw fat, especially raw cow cream, is key to healing). Indeed, the hyperactivity that many children display is, in my opinion, just an instinctive uncoordinated effort to reinforce the physical biological connection between the two hemispheres of the brain. As he was unusually flexible for a seven-year-old boy, we then introduced various yogic positions while listening to Russill Paul's wonderful Bhava or Shabda yogic music. He would continue these exercises and asanas (positions) for many months as his proper neuronal connectivity increased and his unneeded neuronal connections hopefully "disconnected." Of course, most essential to all of this was the introduction of raw fats to allow for this nerve building and proper conduction as well as to help detoxify heavy metals (as heavy metals are raw fat-soluble). Fortunately, the mother supported all the dietary changes (she was aware of many basic useful dietary precautions) and the boy liked the raw veggie juicing, raw cow dairy, and raw egg drinks— a great start. Later we added other special raw food concoctions to speed up the brain connectivity and increase his muscular strength. After just a few weeks, his mother noticed that he started to apologize to people (especially his family), which was unusual for him and a positive sign for us, after he had impulsively "bothered" them.

We continued to treat him with needles, laser, exercises, inert gas combinations, encouraging loving words and diet for about six months. By that time, he was doing right/left brain exercises and yogic positions on his own. His speech was noticeably improved so he could verbally communicate better and his family relations were, while not good, improving. His teachers told me that he was noticeably better and more easily redirected. He was studying better and had started mixing in more with regular classes. This increased his self-confidence and allowed him to feel more in control of his life. He also was able to make friends -the importance of which can not be overestimated. All this was very encouraging, especially to his mother who was also dealing with other challenging life situations. These were the first major improvements she had seen in her son in years, and the fear of things getting worse finally started to subside. His mother kept the boy coming and did well to see that he got the raw fats, did more "brain exercises" and meditated with some aids. The mother also grew spiritually from seeing this situation in a whole new light and this gave her some much needed inspiration and hope. She had been courageous in her raising of this son and now it was rewarding for her to receive some real practical help mixed with metaphysical teasings suggesting the wonderful potentials which awaited her if she kept up this healing path for her and her son (and also, later, her other children).

I believe that one must honor children for choosing to incarnate with difficult Karmic paths that in this case was in many ways, at this young age, harder on the family than on the boy himself. **All the therapy had to be done in a sense that we were encouraging him at a soul level to want to redirect various energies in order to realign his nervous system. The mother eventually approached a place in her "heart-mind" where she could actually be grateful to her son** for allowing her the opportunity for accelerated soul growth and "burning-off" or balancing of Karma by dealing with her son's condition. She was now able to deal with him with not just love and patience, but with healing gratitude and healing dietary/biological knowledge and the implementation of such on both metaphysical and physical levels.

I suspected that if the boy continued with the high fat diet and various daily practices which we had initiated, he would continue to develop and his brain would adapt and develop rapidly as most brain's naturally do if fed raw fats. Remember, cholesterol is the brain's main organic molecule.

Acupuncture can often reduce anxiety levels considerably. Many people find common herbs like Valerian effective as an anxiolytic-sedative due to its evidenced agonistic properties of one of the many types of serotonin receptors (the 5-HT5a receptor) by Guido et al. at the Univ. of Illinois Chicago, Pharmacy Department. (A complicated and well researched plethora of information on herbology exists and has much to offer in most medical areas). Much of my practice is now centered around pediatric anxiety as it is a prevailing symptom in many psychiatric cases and life in general. When I worked with pediatric psychiatric referrals in hospitals, I knew that many of them would benefit from acupuncture treatments to reduce anxiety, stomach/ intestinal discomfort, insomnia, fear, and appetite adjustments. I worry that if the hypothalamus-pituitary- adrenal axis (HPA axis) is continually over stimulated in young children that it may not return to homeostasis (typical regularity) easily. This over-stimulation of the HPA axis results in a sense of over vigilance and defensiveness that is weakening. Anxiety and the HPA axis connection is the subject of much research. Hopefully, we can learn to stop this anxiety driven over stimulation in young children to obviate future problems. Reducing anxiety should be a key goal of all healthcare practitioners.

Research has supported acupuncture's role in treating various psychiatric conditions via its manipulation (increase) of central nervous system hormones like pituitary beta-endorphin(analgesic) and ACTH (anti-inflammation via cortisol), serotonin and noradrenalin(activates descending antinoceptive pathways) as well as urinary MHPG-sulfate (inversely related to schizophrenic severity). Acupuncture can also relieve anxiety by: increasing prominent brain alpha-rhythms, decreasing pain perception, modulating neuropeptide-Y system in the amygdale, and increasing endogenic nocturnal melatonin secretion.1-5 Acupuncture may help obviate the empirically-obvious adverse metabolic changes (increased adiposity and decreased insulin sensitivity) one sees so often with atypical antipsychotics-especially in children.

A concern with many medicines is the detox required after taking the medicine. ADHD medicines especially tend to leave alot of brain residues and the brain can take time to detox as it is **glial-based not lymph-based** in its cleansing mechanism. Raw cream and blueberries empirically allow for chemical binding of many toxins like metals and then excretion. Raw organic nuts (not cashews or peanuts)like walnuts are also significant brain enhancers. **The brain being 60% fat (and half of that is animal fat) demands lots of raw animal fat and raw dairy cream is easiest for most.**

Sadly, it is clear that many cases of ADHD can be traced back to some type of shock or abuse in very early childhood. This shock or abuse does also include perceived shocks, nightmares, past live memories of trauma or violence. At times it can even be a loud noise that shocks the baby and is perceived by the baby as traumatic. It is also often real abuse be it physical or emotional this lifetime. Parents rarely want to consider this but over time many will see that sadly this is empirically true.

1. Hans JS. *ElectroAcupuncture: An alternative to antidepressants for treating affective disease.* J Neuroscience 1986; 29: 79-92

2. Kessler R., et al. *The use of CAM in treating anxiety and depression.* Am Psychiatry 2002; 73: 367-382

3. Mamtani R. et al. *CAM in the treatment of mental health problems.* PsychiatriQ 2001;158:289-294

4. Paolucci D. et al. *Acupuncture and beta-endorphin and ACTH levels.* Lancet. 1979;2:535-536

5. Wu MT et al. *Central nervous pathway for acupuncture stimulation: localization of processing with fMRI.* Radiology. 1999; 21: 133-141

Case #2:

Blindness in an infant

"man's inhumanity to man is so easily seen on a daily basis. The wrong path is to shut down the heart's eyes for this would tell the baby to do likewise."

I was referred a three-month-old baby boy of Asian ancestry. There was visual impairment the extent of which at this young age is hard to diagnose as the eye function is still developing and does not reach adult type strength until nine years of age. It was feared that the child would be functionally blind. There was some eye history in the family with the need for strong glasses. The boy held his head a bit forward as such babies often do which leads to neck problems and malformed sternocleidomastoid (neck) musculature. The weight and skull size appeared to be a bit below average which is not uncommon. Japanese tend to have large cranial and foot width sizes by Western standards and along with their golden skin tone at birth (due to higher bile storage easily reduced with light therapy) and black hair makes for an impressive sight when born. The golden skin tones contrasted with the black hair is beautifully striking to many Westerners.

Fortunately, the baby came to us when he was at an age where eye formation and nerve conduction could still be ameliorated to some degree (many times by a large degree) by a diet high in healing raw fats and very limited carbohydrates, especially complex carbohydrates.

It is difficult to convince many Asian patients them that rice and soy products are particularly damaging in general, but particularly to the eyes. However, with proper readings and a caring approach this parental impediment can often be overcome. Much of the toxic by-products of cooked foods are also imparted to the baby in the mother's milk; thus, the mother had to change her diet. The impaired musculature involved in eyesight is usually improved within a year or so if both electrical stimulation (to acupuncture eye control points) is used and the raw diet is followed by mother and baby. Some also do acupuncture on various traditional eye points located on the limbs and ear. Replicated research studies have shown that these distal eye acu-points do excite the visual cortex. This improvement is easily seen as the child can control his eye movement better and often the two eyes start to move together. This improvement is very encouraging to the parents, but is actually the easiest part of this type problem to ameliorate. The baby boy easily accepted raw cow cream, raw goat milk, raw eggs, avocadoes and enjoyed various beautiful traditional Asian and native American music.

As one can imagine the importance of touch and sound/music is paramount with the visually impaired. It is always an honor for me to be able to work with the parents of such children and to be able to help them augment a child's non-visual senses before the vision improves. Of course, the parents, especially the dominant (main caregiver) parent, must educate and prepare themselves responsibly for such a healing path with scientific knowledge about what the eyes represent, how they function anatomically, of what nerves are composed, how to increase the muscular coordination and strength involved in vision.

The most important factor is that the parents learn to tease or illicit the desire to see from the baby's heart and psyche. The baby has chosen these parents with these DNA characteristics to challenge both him and the parents in a path of accelerated soul growth. The parents cannot control this karmic pattern in total, but they can do much to coax the desire to see from the baby's consciousness. To acknowledge the baby's decision to be born with this challenge and to honor his path and his influence on the parents is important. Many lifetimes of Karma may be "burnt-off" or balanced with wise decisions surrounding the raising and assisting of children.

The thing that is so hard to put into practice is the implications of the understanding that babies live through the parents' sense impressions to some extent. **The child will see through the parents' eyes and the parents' emotional patterns which the baby may actually feel and often see as brightness or darkness even if functionally blind. This sensitivity makes every touch and sound so poignant and special.**

I always encourage such parents to make as much time as possible to train themselves with black goggles or a blinder to approximate a bit what it might be like and how important other sens-es become, and how as the baby grows the reassuring loving words must be heard frequently by such visually impaired babies. Parents must reassess what they are listening to daily on TV or stereo and how they react (verbally and non-verbally) to news and talk. The baby will be absorbing these energies.

Babies will directly tune into parents' sense reactions— even non-verbally. This attunement will help the parents learn how not to be so judgmental and how to control their reactions so that they are not just reacting without independent thought process even when they disagree with something they hear on TV etc.... Of course, this ideally starts during the pregnancy.

Even the way one touches such a baby can have more resonance with practice. All this must also be done with a sense of encouraging the baby non-verbally to want to see. It is important to playfully tease the baby about the fact that he or she is, indeed, missing something that could be seen with their eyes if they would like to turn a little more conscious energy toward the physical eye area. The key point here is to remember that karmic ally the baby has chosen not to see initially and **how the parents see and sense things will directly affect the child's desire to want to see with the eyes.**

Now why would someone not want to see? I usually assume that one does not want to see aspects of suffering and cruelty in the world; man's inhumanity to man is so easily seen on a daily basis. The wrong path is to shut down the heart's eyes for this would tell the baby to do likewise. It does not just about understand the immense beauty in the world and how animals, nature and people can interact and learn to understand and love, but it is also about watching the whole gradual process of transformation through suffering in humanity — ongoing and improving. The goal is not to avoid watching or thinking about tragic events but to watch

One's reactions to such thoughts or news; to understand how to view aspects of war, violence and terrorism as a source for deeper understanding around the concepts of forgiveness and understanding that will lead to more peace and understanding. Of course, exposing oneself and the baby to beauty of all types and letting him sense your enthrallment with beauty will also be of much benefit.

The important mental games that the mother or primary parent figure must learn to do are not difficult or rigid but must be done daily so that the energy field of inquiry is established in the child as early as possible non-verbally before the age of around two. After about two years of age more verbal games become more useful in therapy. The rule-of-thumb is for the mother to ask herself if there is some aspect of her understanding of a relationship in life or even factual information she has received over the years that she would like to see/understand more clearly; to review one's own judgments about people in one's life that have become so fixed; to reevaluate how we see others and learn to be flexible. One can often gain great understanding about oneself from these practices and impart to the baby this energy of flexibility in thinking and reconsideration.

To do all one can do to encourage the child to establish a psychological link in order to see or to desire to see is the most important factor here because proper raw diet, acupuncture, lasers, herbs and scientific vibration therapies can usually ameliorate most physical impairments in infants and is quite easy to implement. I saw the psychological aspects as the dominant root cause of this blindness. In this child's case, we used an eyebright formula (tincture) that we have had good success with in the past. The same as a flower essence can also be potent in a bath. We rarely recommend cooked/boiled herbs anymore (or any cooked food or boiled drink for that matter) as they seem to invoke an immune reaction that stresses the body. We also used audiovisual integration devices (flashing light therapy). I stress the benefit of the use of well-made tuning forks that emit certain frequencies relating to certain frequencies of parts of the body. These vibration therapies are particularly wonderful here because the tuning forks can be felt on the body as well as heard. It is joyous to watch infants reactions to various frequencies and clearly therapeutic. The infant will react with attention when they hear the tuning forks approaching but before the fork is actually touched to their body. Then, as the fork gets closer and touches their body, they often emit this wonderful laughter or some babies start to get sleepy depending on the frequencies of the forks.

We also used movement therapy as this boy got older. By 36 months of age, he was doing fairly rhythmical movements to various sacred music, animal sounds and chanting. This movement must be encouraged daily and initially with the visually impaired one must take the child's arms, legs, waist, head, etc...and manually move them repeatedly with love and visual imaging and then have the baby touch your body as you move rhythmically to sound or to breath. The child can resist various training aspects so, of course, it takes persistence and a strong will, but mostly loving wisdom of what benefits could come by such training. This boy was lucky in that both his mother and father fully participated and the mother was not working and able to devote much time to understanding the deeper concepts of nourishing another. The mother told me that she never knew such a meaningful, interesting lifestyle could be hers and she started studying "tai chi chuan" and yoga in order to learn more about movement, breath and healing touch. She became an inspiration to other mothers who had no idea of what to do with their visually impaired babies. Most mothers love and hope for the best for their children, but this is not in itself sufficient for healing in many cases. (Mothers in the USA are at times much easier to work with than mothers in Japan because the rigid, fixed way of thinking in Japan leaves little room for self-empowerment, metaphysical thinking and doing something independently).

We treated the mother and the baby under the pyramid together to enhance the resonance between them and allow for more direct attunement to their own subtle bodies. The mother learned to use tuning forks and crystals activated by cold laser on the baby and herself. She became proficient at meditating in the presence of the baby and learned to control her own thought forms and emotions in a more loving way and the boy learned much from these practices. This boy could see functionally with strong glasses by age six, but because of all his training and spiritual growth, had developed other special senses and abilities that will make him stand out from others over the years. He moved gracefully and was of considerable coordination and refinement. I suspect that as the optic nerve continues to develop through the teen years, the boy's vision will continue to improve.

Case #3:

Tinnitus/ auditory resonance disorder

Skeletal bones are the acoustic instruments that conduct sound.

This was a 28-year old female patient with no major medical history. She was thin, attentive, pretty, and had a comparatively good cooked diet (very low in fried foods and high in raw fish and vegetables). Her main complaint was the sensations or sounds she would get in her head once a week or so that she described as auditory speeding up and necessitating her lying down until the "spell" past (usually 20 minutes). She would hear sped up indistinguishable sounds that disorientated her. She had no seizures, loss of consciousness or memory and was mentally present during these episodes. It was a scary feeling for her, as she had no idea what it was. It was a bit paralyzing emotionally for her and clearly debilitating.

I have seen similar symptoms mostly in clients who came from very traditional close-knit cultures outside the USA. It is an interesting disorder that could originate as a result of emotional suppression common in certain traditional inflexible cultures: to have something within the consciousness that is not communicated; something perhaps that everyone knows in the village or in the family but no one talks about. This suppression may have been a survival mechanism yet, on the positive side, one of the choices for some people to be attracted to a more open and freely expressive society such as the States. This trend reflects what I believe is actually a "genetic shift" in priorities; opting for truth over harmony in order to work out the deeper issues and is an important lesson for many people in this life. Thus, many head to Western countries, especially the States. Although much of my experience in treating clients faced with this challenge has been in Asia, I suspect that people from many other traditional cultures might experience similar afflictions.

Physically, this suppression often manifests as a short period (a few seconds to an hour) in which everything speeds up in the brain or sounds are distorted inside the head. It is fearful for most as it is rarely discussed and rarely balanced. A few patients have been able to have MRIs during such an episode and activity in parts of the auditory complex was seen. (This same phenomena of cerebral auditory excitation in an MRI has been evidenced during auditory hallucinations in schizophrenics i.e. they are actually hearing voices.) However, the point I stress is that this can be seen as a healing function of the body. It is below the realm of even a minor seizure yet disturbing to the person since it is so strange.

I see it as an intercommunication and resonance throughout the brain. When the resonance occurs, various components from one side can communicate with the other. There are ways to correct this but it helps to see it is part of the healing process and not something to be feared but experienced in a positive light. These are energies that are there to resolve excommunicated issues. Once I explain this to my clients they are relieved, and they slowly learn to sit and experience these episodes in a positive healing light. Thus, the episodes eventually become shorter and less intense. Just having someone tell them that what they are feeling and hearing is not as uncommon or strange as they think allows for a healing shift in consciousness to set in. The fear is reduced and healing can begin.

This client initially called me when she sensed an episode coming on, and I stayed with her on the phone until it was over or largely subsided. Often it is just that one time with someone knowledgeable there to support them, even over the phone, which makes all the difference in the world. There are also various meditative and visualization techniques that she learned to do during the episodes that greatly accelerated the healing process.

Now, again, various forms of energy work, especially certain types of acupuncture with geomantic technologies and specific meditative practices, can greatly enhance many healing processes to raise the energy in a gentle and clear way for most patients take time. This patient would totally relax under the pyramid and could feel the cold lasers at distal points from where they were focused on the body. She could feel the needle energy sensations and other frequency devices all along the acupuncture pathways (meridians) if they were stimulated properly. Tuning into the physical body, being aware of it as an important way of sourcing and working with these energies and recirculating them is valuable.

Sometimes this accelerated right-left brain resonance is com-plicated when there are insufficient energies in the brain which I assume result in fragile neuronal connections between right and left-brain. I surmise this from empirical evidence by judging which patient "attacks" can be triggered by a sufficient disturbance of an

electromagnetic nature, of an emotional nature, even a geopathic nature e.g., Hartman and Curry lines,* resulting in a push over the edge so to speak in which these brain patterns become a powerful resonance. Therefore, a high raw fat diet is necessary to reinforce nerves (as nerves are high in fat) and allow for a more efficient less stressful nerve conduction. Raw butter, raw cream, avocadoes, raw oils and raw meat fats are all helpful in different ways.

Many patients have an impaired nervous system which can be overwhelmed with feelings of sadness, helplessness and apathy that can easily lead to suicide or just increased levels of fear and impo-tence. However, one must view this as a chance to heal. One can always view the cup as half-empty/half full or realize that one needs a bigger cup. There are always interesting implications when one accepts the self-responsibility often lacking in the healing process. When one chooses to accept self-responsibility and speed up one's Karma it truly is a fascinating and challenging thing to watch unfold. Holding the context here as to perceiving how to deal with a challenge in life makes all the difference in the world. One must ask what is good about it, what is resonated about how one can change and so on. Usually we have to use subtle energy devices in the clinic to facilitate all healing as this brings to the surface some of the difficult underlying energies to which one must not be succumbed but ask what is the cause of one's fear. **If one finds the capacity to surrender, to awaken the energy, to welcome it, to see how it can change oneself etc., there can be value that is established from this. As the energy is able to create a new resonant pattern within the brain, there can be a higher consciousness or awakening.**

The purpose of bringing these new energies into the patient's consciousness is to look at the very nature of consciousness, fear, underlying issues as well as speed-up some of the karma involved. This patient told me that she had made many positive changes in her life but when the "sad/sound attack" (as she called these "attacks") happened, she took it as a sign that she was not doing the right thing or that she was getting sicker somehow.

Over four months this patient's "sound attacks" (as she called them) decreased to a much less intense level and usually only lasted 1-5 minutes. After six months, she reported that she had not had an episode in one month! She was greatly relieved and this encouraged her to try other subtle energy modalities and consider new ways of thinking. She took up photography and started writing memories of her life in her native country and the States and all the things she liked and disliked growing-up now that she could see things from a fresh distant overseas perspective.

(Hartmann and Curry lines refer to lines of electro-magnetic radiation coming from the earth running both north-south and east-west. Some are of a positive charge and others of a negative charge. Areas where certain lines cross are called "stress zones" or geopathic zones" and are thought by many to have negative effects on Human biology. These were researched in Germany in the 1920's. Something as simple as moving one's bed a foot or two can often be very therapeutic.)

Case 4:

Depression and Anxiety

The thought of suicide is a great consolation: by means
of it one gets successfully through many a bad night.
—Friedrich Nietzsche

     This was a 35-year-old female patient who had become un-
motivated, bored and depressed over the past few years since moving to the USA. After much discussion, I suspected that she was
incapable of dealing with the breaking of the law of inertia in her
life i.e., a body at rest tends to stay at rest— she was stuck energetically and could not get moving. Often an incident triggers
a gradual emotional shift into fear and one lacks the appropriate
emotion such as anger to initiate change. Anger can be a great cata-
lytic energy when seen as a reaction to or strategy against fear. We
started this patient on a simple exercise of staying in motion during
the day. Dancing, walking, anything so that she was moving consciously and trying to feel her body move as opposed to not actually
consciously acknowledging her body movements. This movement
had to be done for a set time daily and during this time she had
to watch carefully for her reactions when other energies become
present such as a phone call, someone talking to her etc.... When
these "invasive" energies happened, she would pay close attention
to see if any paralyzing energies showed up in her to stop her for
a moment and create a defensive reaction. To be able to acknowledge an area where change needs to occur is a wonderful starting

point. This patient chose to watch her reactions when the phone rang (which is a common trigger point for many people). She could easily feel her stomach becoming a bit tight upon hearing the first ring and deciding whether to answer the phone. She chose to touch her stomach at these times and relax, breathe, and wait a few rings and answer in a more relaxed state-of-mind. Initially, she decided to run to the phone with a forced laugh to overcome this subtle fear reaction. This, however, just sent a contradictory energy out to the universe. The point is not to override a real feeling or reaction but to change it to one of a more positive vibration. This adjustment is often done by first moving to a place of emotional neutrality and from there to a more positive feeling. These initial reactions which lead to no motion or a lack of forward movement in life must be changed before other larger more positive life changes can evolve. After the phone reactions were dealt with (in this case it took three months for some improvement and nine months before she could feel neutrality or lack of emotion upon hearing the phone ring) other common essential daily areas of life were approached with a similar behavioral methodology.

My concern with this patient was that somewhere down the line as the changes became more challenging, her old passive do-nothing habit patterns would reassert themselves and she would side with the familiar motionless energies, which told her that it is just easier to be complacent and not initiate deeper changes.

Depression is the most common psychiatric illness in The States. About 40% of those who actually do seek medical help do not respond to conventional pharmacological intervention and the dropout rate is about 15%. One study (Luo et al., 1998) found acupuncture to as effective as amitriptyline for depressive symptoms.

Patients, in a study by Yang et al., 1994, evidenced better outcomes with respect to somatization and cognitive process disturbances than those on medication. As with the first case study, acupuncture has been evidenced in neurotransmitter and hormone modification. Even though lack of serotonin has not been proven to be a cause of depression, many people do feel better with longer cellular exposure times. This is the same with many drugs like amphetamine stimulants given for ADHD patients—- one feels better on them, but this does not mean that your body is biologically deficient without them. Acupuncture can increase cerebral serotonin levels.

(repeat from case #1: Research has supported acupuncture's role in treating various psychiatric conditions via its manipulation (increase) of central nervous system hormones like pituitary beta-endorphin(analgesic) and ACTH (anti-inflammation via cortisol), serotonin and noradrenalin(activates descending antinoceptive pathways) as well as urinary MHPG-sulfate (inversely related to schizophrenic severity). Acupuncture can also relieve anxiety by: increasing prominent brain alpha-rhythms, decreasing pain perception, modulating neuropeptide-Y system in the amygdale, and increasing endogenic nocturnal melatonin secretion.1 Acupuncture may help obviate the empirically-obvious adverse metabolic changes (increased adiposity decreased insulin sensitivity) one sees so often with atypical antipsychotics-especially in children).

As with many cases of depression, I assumed that there were insufficient strains of bacteria evolving in the small intestine. I have seen frequent empirical/clinical evidence that depression can be ameliorated if there are **adequate bacteria interacting in the small intestine to directly produce numerous factors like hormones (dopamine) as well as signals (various peptides) to the brain to produce many neurotransmitters like serotonin etc (most of which is produced in the small intestine)** and to prevent harmful chemicals from thriving in the intestines.

Some Lactobacilli and Bifido produce anti-anxiety GABA, some Escherichia produce norepinephrine, and some Bacillus can produce dopamine and Streptococcus can make serotonin. . These are many of the happy chemicals people are seeking their whole life. Small intestine research is difficult to do due to access inconvenience. Large intestine research and the incredibly complex symbiosis, quorum-sensing and signaling of trillions of microbes is still overwhelming. Many tribal cultures have cultivated aged meats, dairy and cheeses to counter depressed feelings and to keep their peoples happy. As I have seen clinically, organic dirt has more healthful bacterial strains and are the quickest path to reversing depression and overall healing and have no ill side-effects. Only fecal transplants will help some people who are too afraid to eat bacteria.

This patient, after many months of coaxing and light-hearted joking, finally sat down with me and together we had a tiny bite of organic hamburger meat that I had aged for six weeks. She bravely held her nose and downed a tiny bite. The patient felt a pleasant happy feeling within twenty min-utes and it lasted for about five hours. This one positive experience with encouraging support was all she needed to set her on a road to health. Her reaction and thought process was typical-she thought the idea of the aged or spoiled meats was disgusting, but the pleasant feeling she received after eating one piece gave her intuitive and physical confirmation that this was the way to go. She had been able to reduce her anti-depressant dosage from 60mg down to 10 mg over 6 months prior to the aged meats by receiving acupuncture, spinal manipulation ("tui-na") and doing coordinated anal/vaginal sphincter breathing.

Another consideration with my Japanese female clients, in general, is that they are raised in an atmosphere where acceptance is so important. I have observed over many years that many Asian females are inherently ultra-sensitive to others thoughts. What people in the West always see the moment they view certain ethnic faces for the first few seconds is the ethnicity of the face (although many can't distinguish Japanese from Chinese morphology), the lineage, and this is sensed by many people and can create an inner barrier. Thus one must acknowledge their own intuitive sensitivities as being raised in a certain society, like Japan (but many others also) with the inherent subtle undermining of a woman's sense of value inherent there and the suppressing of so many feelings and thought processes which must be controlled if a woman is to act without resentment and rebellion as is required in Japan for the sake of a harmonious society or whatever erroneous reason the male dominated powers that be mandate.

Now, many Japanese living in the West, particularly the States, have logically seen that the support that is given at both the psychological level and physical level is superior now with the world they have created overseas in the West. This patient was the same. She loved all the new opportunities and freedom here in the States. She appreciated the high standard of living, lack of crowds, relative low rents (or more space for the same rent) and access to nature. She had taken advantage of the health clubs and holistic supermarkets. After a while, however, she became too discouraged and antidepressants and alcohol did not help much. What is hard to shift is the sense of belonging regardless of a happy family or work-life here in the States. Being part of a group is powerfully brought in (perhaps even through the genetics) generation after generation in Japan. This group energy has been key in Japan's international domination phase of their karma. The Japanese sense of unity and international interconnectivity has created powerful world energies that create admiration but also fear.

These formidable energies, whether good or bad, inherently healthy or unhealthy, whether they are inherently supporting overseas Japanese goals and aims in this life for independence, support and understanding is immaterial. They are still powerful energies that may well have been within the genetic lineage for a long time. Breaking away from this one way or another is an important attribute for many Japanese living in the States. It is part of their karmic attraction to the West and ability to move out of Japan.

Considering various ways for themselves to break away from this Japanese consciousness is a powerful adjunct to each person's soul therapy. Exploring one's own creativity in this area is important. Some things that people decide to look into or work with may seem at first silly or irrelevant to others but that does not matter. What is important is the idea of bringing into form some sense of support for making this shift for making really a right turn in the evolution of this energy. Those able to make such a shift have much to offer to the world and especially to other Japanese. This new vitality and dynamic thinking is easily perceived by those with enough firsthand knowledge of Japanese in Japan and those abroad who could adapt. The difference is striking and beautiful to behold.

Much of the karma that Japan has incurred with various aspects of harm to others is coming to a place of deeper self-consciousness, awareness and understanding. As it relates to the Japanese sense of national identity, dealing with an honest approach to history will absolutely require a new perspective. A perspective completely outside the Japanese consciousness in order to see and understand itself is needed. For this reason now many Japanese individuals consciously and subconsciously are preparing to become more independent and moving abroad is, for many, an essential step in obtaining this independence. Understanding and working with this more consciously is difficult because one often receives the messages at an emotional level or internal level.

(One newer mode of shifting consciousness in Japan is stand-up comedy. As Japanese learn to laugh at themselves, they learn to break the mold. After all, Japanese children are told over and over again not to do this or that or someone will laugh at them. This is how manners are taught. Still, the ability for Japanese to appreciate self-deprecation and actually laugh at themselves is key to healing and that which is so sorely needed. The United States has much to share and teach in this respect).

REFERENCES

International Conference on Unsolved Problems of Noise and Fluctuations in Physics& Biology: Maryland NIH lectures: 2002 "Can Intrinsic Fluctuations Increase Efficiency in Neuronal Information Processing" Dr. H. Liljenstrom. "Stochastic Growth of Proteome Complexity due to Evolution" Dr. V. Kuznetsov

Hans JS. *ElectroAcupuncture:An alternative to antidepressants for treating affective disease.* J Neurosci 1986; 29: 79-92

Kessler R., et al. *The use of CAM in treating anxiety and depression.* Am Psych 2002; 73: 367-382

Luo H et al. *Clinical research on the therapeutic effect of acupuncture with depression.* Psych Neurosci. 1998;52:338-340

Mamtani R. et al. *CAM in the treatment of mental health problems.* PsychiatriQ 2001;158:289-294

Roschke J. et al. The benefit of whole body acupuncture in major depression. J Affect Disord. 2000; 57:73-80

Yang X. et al. *Clinical observation on needling points in treating mental depression.* J Trad Chin Med. 1994; 14: 14-18

Case 5:

Chronic Pain

The tragedy of life is what dies inside a man while he lives.

-Albert Schweitzer

A 35-year-old female was referred to my clinic by a local pediatrician. Her main complaint was chronic severe pain in the arch area of both feet. The Western diagnosis was plantar tendon fasciitis. Walking short distances was painful but standing more than a few minutes in one place or walking any distance was unbearable. She had been to many doctors who practiced various forms of Western medicine to no avail. All tests had shown no abnormalities with nerve and muscle anatomy or function, and bone formation was normal. She had had surgery on the tendon of one foot with no amelioration in pain. The usual trigger-point laser therapy also did not help this patient. I have found that certain lasers are more effective than 1% Lidocain on trigger points. Longer acting local anesthetics are probably toxic to some degree and as inflammatory causes at trigger points are not evidenced, strong steroid use is questionable.(As an important aside, fibromyalgia type pain and weakness usually responds very well to acupuncture and raw foods)

The patient had been taking various opiate-based medicine. One problem with opiate-based medicines is that aside from constipation and addiction, these drugs tend to imbalance the HPG (hypothalamus-pituitary-gonadal) hormonal axis which results in sex steroids (testosterone, estrogens, and progesterone) deficiency called hypogonadism. Decreased energy and sex drive/ability, weight gain, depression, and irregular menstruation result in many people. Naloxone, which is an opiate receptor antagonist with a very high affinity for "mu" opiod receptors, has also been used off label for pain control along with opiates. Perhaps this seems counter-intuitive but how many medicines actually work physiologically (always ignoring the spiritual and subtle influences) is often not understood. The end result is seen and that is enough. **Perhaps low doses of naloxone cause a compensatory cellular signaling that increases the number of opiate receptors or natural body pain killers output.**

(For suspected heroin addicts lying unconscious where I worked in various S. E. Asian clinics, naloxone was a mainstay. We were supposed to check pulse, oxygen levels, and blood-sugar and then administer naloxone. Eventually, one saw that the older clinicians just gave naloxone directly as it was a detox center and most of the patients were addicts. Often they were found outside unconscious. Once naloxone was injected into the muscle of an addict about to die from respiratory arrest, they would regain con-sciousness before our eyes. If there was no recovery after a minute, another 2mg (up to 10 mg usually) was injected. Giving naloxone to addicts to carry with them is still controversial but will eventually become more accepted. I suspect it saves lives temporarily but it also decreases fear of death by overdose and leads to more risky behavior i.e., more than the excessively risky normal behavior of many addicts. There are also heroin addicts who use more prudently and function normally at work and home. There is considerable evidence to support that electroacupuncture at body points is also particularly effective in alleviating the withdrawal syndrome in heroin addicts (Zheng et al., 2005). The neurochemical and be-havioral evidence of research has shown that acupuncture's role in suppressing the reinforcing effects of abused drugs takes place by modulating mesolimbic dopamine neurons (Kim et al., 2005; Fu-kuda et al., 2004). Also, several brain neurotransmitter systems such as serotonin, opioid and amino acids including GABA have been implicated in the modulation of dopamine release by acupunc-ture. These results provided clear evidence for the biological effects of acupuncture.) **When one is revived with nalaxone it feels awful (but alive)!**

The first thing that struck me when the patient walked in was the lack of connectivity between her body parts. She was not lanky or falling over herself but she seemed to have little sense of what I call physicality. She was alert, depressed, intelligent and sincere. Her pulses, in Oriental terminology, were "choppy mixed with wiry" and very interesting indicating, in general, poor blood circulation somewhere. Her spleen/pancreas pulse was excessive. Although many patients have a poor spleen/pancreas pulse as they eat cooked foods (necessitating the pancreas and liver to produce more enzymes which deplete their other production capacities after many years). She had no lung history or present lung symptoms, but her lung pulse was the weakest comparatively. This weak lung pulse was interesting as the lung is considered the most connected/external organ and any loss of sense of connectivity to Earth and physicality can often be read in the lung pulse. She drank excessive amounts of water daily and liked green tea. Her diet was average i.e., cooked foods but not excessively junky by U.S. standards. She also had a sort of childlike, innocent quality about her which I see more commonly in foreigners i.e. non-USA.

She socialized little and her childhood had been sad as it was dominated by abuse by parents who were life-long addicts, criminals while maintaining professional businesses and this shadowed the rest of her life. She was also clinically a narcissist. Her main complaint was pain, and pain and nerves, being fat based, necessitate raw fat again- biology shows the way to heal again!

There is considerable empirical evidence and research supporting acupuncture's role in pain control. Dr Huey Lee et al at the University of Medicine New Jersey used brain imagery to indicate that acupuncture can influence pain perception, reduce the feeling of pain or even raise pain thresholds. Also, Yun-Kyoung Yim et al. did research in South Korea's Dunson Hospital suggesting acupuncture can reduce inflammation and regulates immune activity in collagen induced arthritis via numerous pathways. Acupuncture therapeutically reduced levels of cytokines and antibodies (Il-6, INF, IgG, IgM) in patients with RA (rheumatoid arthritis). Research has supported acupuncture's role in treating various pain conditions via its manipulation (increase) of central nervous system hormones like pituitary beta-endorphin (analgesic) and ACTH (anti-inflammation via cortisol), serotonin and noradrenalin (activates descending antinoceptive pathways). Very impressive indeed!

We treated her using acupuncture and various inert gas combinations She usually fell asleep when being treated which is usual as she was always a bit wired, generally did not sleep deeply and found it hard to relax.

She was interested in my questions and thoughts regarding his body and personal history. She talked about his lack of coordination or proper nervous/muscular training. The first thing I started her on was reconnecting her right and left brain communication with the same exercises on which we start children with various right-left brain imbalances (attention disorders, coordination problems, certain speech problems). An example of these exercises would be having both arms extended and doing circles in opposite directions simultaneously or right leg and left arm doing opposite movements at the same time. Such seemingly simple exercises are initially very difficult for many but quickly establish new nerve paths in the brain and result in more coordination physically; it does take a few months for most people, as they do not repeat the exercises enough. These physical movement exercises became more complex as she mastered the more simple ones. She enjoyed doing these and regaining a sense of self through physical movement. A basic but essential step in self-empowerment. She was impressed with himself when she could finally do the basic yoga lotus position "padmasana" but not the valuable headstands like "shirhsasana"-one of the most healing asana or positions). We also talked about why she would choose to incarnate in a body with these abusive parents. The ability to analyze the good points of one's karmically chosen family and life experiences in a karmic light is essential for all patients' healing. Many patients are open to this practice and idea when it is presented to them in a matter-of-fact way.

I hoped that she could eventually come to and work through a point of resentment toward others in her life for not helping her become more coordinated when she was a youth obviously poor at sports and similar physical activities which she had wanted to do. Why she had not been able to karmically attract someone to aid her in her childhood when it would scar her for life at some level? After much thinking and questioning, she did work through this resentment, and this facilitated the process of forgiveness. Eventually, after many more months, she could actually appreciate her trials in life and pondered what advantage there was to her present situation and what special events life would show her once she allowed herself to heal.

She had to work on appreciating her body, soul and spirit as it was, is and could be. She had to learn not to judge herself, but to love herself for who she was and would be. She eagerly started the raw diets in increments and bought a juicer right away. She was open to the raw foods to a point. She started on avocados, cold-pressed olive oil, vegetable juicing, but was leery about the raw proteins (meats, eggs, organs etc...). It was a good first effort. I continued to stress the importance of raw proteins as cooked proteins produce a variety of 20 different toxic heterocyclic amines and lead to aging, stress and terminal imbalances. I had advised her to be aware of any digestive disorders that may manifest in a subtle manner such as heaviness as opposed to pain or diarrhea.

This patient also had to deal with a dislike/fear of bacteria, bugs, dirt and disorder in general which may have been due to the depression or merely an attempt to control aspects of life for a sense of safety. She needed to "loosen-up" as they say and allow herself to get messy sometimes without minding it. Initially, many practices I encouraged her to do would go against her nature and she would find them disagreeable. The key point is to be able to do various new things without feeling discomfort or disgust as opposed to just forcing oneself to do something for the sake of doing it.

As I felt she was so disconnected to Mother Earth's healing energy, I had her walk in bare feet on grass or bury her feet in the dirt, sand, mud etc... As her sense of physicality and her awareness of her connection to Mother Earth grew, I surmised that her feet would be nourished and her pain eradicated.

As always one must consider past life abuses that most people need to deal with by asking forgiveness of those they abused in past lives or forgive those who abused them. Many psychosomatic pains are also relieved by this practice (perpetrator-victim karma is often repeated with reverse roles). One can learn to feel what aspect of their "consciousness" is feeling the pain that is perceived as being physical.

She continued this conscious Earth-walking practice, which eventually led her to being able to meditate as she walked. She could feel that as she breathed in, she was actually absorbing/accepting various vibrational energies from the Earth. One day she will break through the illusion that it is actually her breathing independently of universal energies/spirit.

References

Fukuda F, Shinbara H, Yoshimoto K, Ozaki A, et al. Alterations in the function of cerebral dopaminergic and serotonergic systems following electroacupuncture and moxibustion applications: possible correlates with their antistress and psychosomatic actions. *Neurochem Res* (2004) 29:: 283–93

Kim SH, Lee YK, Kim TH, et al. Effect of acupuncture on behavioral hyperactivity and dopamine release in the nucleus accumbens in rats sensitized to morphine. *Neurosci Lett* (2005;) 387:: 17–21

Zeng X, Lei L, Lu Y, Wang Z. Treatment of heroinism with acupuncture *J Tradit Chin Med* (2005) 25:: 166–70

.

Pregnancy:
nurturing the instinctive raw
diet in the baby and toddler

"…in the preparation before conception when the couple is trying to attract an appropriate soul to reincarnate through them." book quote

A 28-year-old female patient complained of low back pain and having migraines 2-3 times weekly for the past 20 years. The patient was three months pregnant. I always verify the expected date of delivery (EDD) with the physician or midwife. Many times I have been told the wrong EDD based on erroneous patient information or a wrong calculation by a midwife based on the patient's misinformation. I am often asked to induce labor if a pregnancy is post-term. The problem is that many patients and midwives tell me that the patient is post-term when they really are not late at all. Increasing oxytocin levels is easy in most cases with just acupunc-ture. However, if the baby is not "overdue" and artificially induced via acupuncture or pitocin, there is a greatly increased chance of needing a Caesarian section if the patient is not dilated enough.

She claimed no medical history aside from migraines (which usually improve **gradually** with acupuncture and spinal manipulation treatments) but upon pulse palpation diabetic type pulses (Chinese pulse diagnosis) and a weak kidney area were clear. Upon inquiring about her diabetic pulses, she said that her mom was diabetic, but that she was not. I explained to her that her pulses suggest that her pancreas is already overly stressed due to her carbohydrate abuse, and that her insulin would gradually become impotent and excessive. In addition, the pancreas having to work overtime to produce more enzymes to help her digest cooked foods was exacerbating the situation. She was overweight, alert, intelligent, very tired, and pretty with vibrant skin. Her diet was cooked foods with a lot of snacks and deficient in all nutrients. She seemingly had little idea of how she was nutritionally abusing herself or her baby. She had minimal consciousness of the reality of pregnancy on a spiritual level, but she was pregnant and this opened up all sorts of access ways.

Although she had not prepared spiritually or physically for the pregnancy, she still had time to do so and avert potential (based on her poor pulse readings and family history) some problems in the child's birth and development. After a lot of readings to orientate her towards the reality of the toxicity of cooked foods as well as the spiritual/theosophical teachings on the subtle bodies and the mother/fetal connections (and a lot of enthusiastic encouragement), she willingly started improving her diet by adding raw fats and thinking about reducing carbohydrates and not cooking her meats as thoroughly. She started to think about how she was responsible for her child's health in formation and how what she ate and felt now was forming the baby's nervous system, organs and glands etc...that would set the stage for life.

Our sessions revealed a woman addicted to media and words— a passive way of not experiencing life first hand. She was surprised to hear her lifestyle described as an addiction. We talked about how significant it was to regain self-empowerment as soon as possible in this and other areas in her life. It turned out that she was indeed addicted to TV and perhaps irrelevant talk in general. She moved the large TV out of the main room as a compromise to my encouraging her to throw it out or give it away. She was always willing to consider what I suggested. Since she was pregnant and her Oriental pulse diagnosis worrisome, I pushed her more quickly and urgently than I normally would have pushed someone with her background and lack of consciousness towards health and meta-physics. She initially responded wonderfully. Even though I am sure she thought I was too persistent and repetitive in my encour-agement, she, like many people, responded well when approached with facts and sincerity.

We treated her low back pain and migraines along with treat-ments appropriate for her pancreatic and kidney imbalances. There is some research on acupuncture's role in relieving migraine pain available on line (aside from clinical-based empirical evidence). The brain has many potent pain modulators including serotonin, GABA (gamma amino butyric acid), and beta-endorphin. ACTH (adrenal corticotrophin hormone) and beta-endorphin are two neurotransmitters which are secreted together by the pituitary gland after receiving noxious pain stimuli. Many patients lack the raw fat and amino acids to produce enough hormones in general so dietary concerns are essential. Other patients genetically produce varying amounts of hormones, neurotransmitters, enzymes and everything else. Again, diet must be considered.

"Cupping" is a common technique that is known in many countries. I have seen "vacuum sucking cup" technique done in Africa, Europe, and Asia. Some of my Israeli friends who I knew in Asia were familiar with this cupping technique that they called "bonkers." In cupping, one, to put it simply, applies cups to the skin and this forms a vacuum effect. It is commonly done on the back for coughs and lung ailments but also helps some types of pain. Skin surface certainly produces various reactions and this can at times be very helpful but for some individuals it is just too much stress. Cupping accelerates the fluid movement through the lymph thus producing greater toxicity and reaction if sufficient lymph drainage is not provided in the clinic. Heavy metal contamination can sometimes be exacerbated and create more harm than good. I often wondered why so many patients reacted with difficulty to strong "fire" cupping techniques used in Asia (but like many precious understandings, rarely seen or taught in the West) and finally, when I started doing lymph drainage after the cupping (again not taught much in Oriental medical schools in The States) things improved quickly. The neck/head area lymph nodes drain into the subclavian venous system.. The patient should be taught how to do simple drainage techniques on themselves and everyone in their family. Basics like deep massage and jumping may help a little but scientifically a vibration machine set at 5hz for five minutes is the most effective and equal to about an hour on a trampoline. Raw coconut cream and pineapple is the best lymph food known- especially before the scientific detox bath(105 degrees fahrenheit for 90 minutes). Many cases of lymph problems have been healed with these simple techniques and now that low deuterium water is available most diseases could be healed.

Her migraines were reduced by half within three months. As her migraines abated, she was greatly relieved and she quit her Amitriptyline . She continued to improve but weight issues, poor diet and pulses persisted. We discussed the reality of her genetics and the fact that each generation sees thirty new DNA mutations called SNPs (which if on a gene could cause new imbalances*) and the fact that her child also would most likely develop many imbalances as had almost everyone in her immediate and extended family. We discussed what the pancreas does physically and how that relates to the feeling of sweetness in life and how many people substitute refined foods for a lack of real sweetness in life. She responded well to the acupuncture treatments along with spinal manipulations, lasers, crystals and magnets on critical points to awaken the mother/baby connection. This new way of thinking was a big step for her.

However, she was pregnant, and this opened up numerous access paths to her consciousness, which the baby would assist us in over the next few months. She gradually realized that she could help initiate a break in the genetic signaling of illness in her family and inspire others around her.

It later came to me that maybe she would benefit from an awakening of her intuition. Somewhere along the way, she seemed to have lost touch with her intuition. I always intuited that I could be pushing her too fast and too far and that it might scare her away in that I sensed a deep seeded fear in her regarding certain spiritual aspects of our healing sessions. I thought that these fears were probably based in some childhood events that might be called extrasensory. I have seen that many patients, as children, have had visions and hearings from subtle energy levels that produced natural quick reactions into fear and, with no one to explain these happenings to them, they became stagnant and anxious and shut down such potentials. I sensed this in this patient and was constantly debating what to tell her or not tell her to awaken her intuition and allow for more conscious contact from her baby. I settled on an approach where I would instill a deep sense of relaxation in her during the treatments and this would allow for a chance of communication with her higher self. Various crystals activated with various lasers seem to have a wonderful effect on activating dreaming in a significant way.

This approach eventually did have its desired effect, as she was at times able to receive messages in her dreams. However, she eventually became confused by all this new information and did not, understandably, have the courage to integrate it in her life properly. She started to express anxiety about all the new knowledge she had received. She could not seize her karmic imperative of fully accepting her responsibility in her role of forming the baby's physical body in a more healthful way.

This rejection of our progress up to this point was probably, in part, a result of her less than ideal self-image and lack of self-love. There was some part in her that resented the pregnancy and the fact that she was not being supported as much as she deserved to be. There was also some deep fear around her connecting to her own fetal energies which were not conscious. We discussed the idea of soul mate and ideal partner. I suggested to her that the true soul mate may just be a human's subconscious desire to be consciously united with their own higher-self. We may be looking to complete ourselves with an aspect of our spirit that is there at some level but erroneously consciously perceived to be separate from ourselves. Humans may well consciously acknowledge this desire as a longing to be fulfilled by another.

We put her on a meditation program where she would make a conscious effort to contact her baby boy in the womb by thinking of the beauty of nature at least twice a day for fifteen minutes. We decided that the best times would be upon awakening and before sleeping. Hopefully, this would lead to more frequent contact between mom and son off and on throughout the day. Now, this type of contact does come naturally or intuitively to many mothers, but in some this instinct must be nurtured and carefully developed. This type practice can awaken deeper levels of consciousness in both mother and baby and should be continued throughout childhood. The mother learns to direct her consciousness to the child and to share positive energies with the child. The child will very gradually learn that his own higher subtle body energies can be used for his own healing; his own strengthening and do not have to be pulled into areas that the parents are unconsciously attracted to. The mother had to pay particular attention to what she was worrying about all day long as these energies would be telling the child that one draws one's energy from others, from outside sources, from affairs of the world — this is not true. As the mother learns to draw energy from her own inner self, the child will also learn this balance. I felt that this type of practice was particularly important for this mother/son as I sensed that the proper attention to raw foods would not continue. Therefore, by imparting this type of awareness to her son, he could potentially learn to use his subtle energies to heal himself despite challenging DNA and poor diet.

Potentially the awareness of one's subtle body energies offers greater importance than diet. These energies can be developed later in life but it is potentially easier and more far reaching to start as close to conception as possible; ideally, in the preparation before conception when the couple is trying to attract an appropriate soul to reincarnate through them .

She was, by that time in her development, already full-term. Her blood pressure had risen and fallen over the pregnancy, but during the last month her pressure was fine. Her birth was not a Caesarian as feared (Cesarian babies have a significant disadvantage of being exposed to less bacteria and thus prone to various problems), and the last trimester had been pretty much pain free. The little boy was born healthy by Western medical standards. However, the quick superficial, but useful, checks that infants receive at birth can do nothing to indicate to the parents developmental problems that are likely to occur as the brain, glands and organs develop and integrate in a poor, albeit subtle, manner as the child grows. Even the lack of raw fats during the gestation period will hamper the nervous system (including the brain's) development to its fuller potential. I suspected that a diet including toxic baby formulas and a lack of raw fats would activate this baby's DNA predisposition toward various inherited imbalances starting with the condition of being overweight as a toddler. The child was overweight by the age of two and lacked coordination.

The valuable role that viruses play in cleaning the body and manipulation of DNA is misunderstood. Many influenza vaccines in the USA sometimes still contain a mercury-based preservative called thimerasol in trace amounts or larger doses in the influenza vaccine which, if injected, is very hard for the body to detoxify (as opposed to dental filling mercury which is more problematic if hot oral liquid allows mercurial gases to penetrate). Adjuvants are substances added to some vaccines (especially non-live or inactivated) to augment the humoral (antibody), cytokine and T-cell immune response. The complexity of immunity must not be underestimated and much is not understood. Adjuvants are generally immune potentiators or antigen delivery systems. Alum (Aluminum salts hydroxide and phosphate) has been the main adjuvant approved for human use. In multiple vaccines together in one shot, the level of aluminum is not prudent. Much research is done looking for effective new adjuvants to increase the immune response to numerous microbes and cancer. There are now in the USA vaccines against 30 diseases with about many more in design. These vaccines will become cleaner, more targeted and adjuvants specificity toward stimulating antibody or antibody isotypes formation over cell-mediated or T-cell subsets immunity will become more accurately engineered.

A well-known publicized case is the Polio immunizations, which contained the simian (monkey) virus SV40 that is known to cause cancer. Supposedly, the virus was removed from polio vaccines after 1963 but this is still unclear even as of January of 1997 when the NIH, the FDA and the CDC met in Bethesda, Maryland joined by scientists from around the world. (Between 1961 and 1976, there were three manufacturers of oral poliovirus vaccine in the United States. In the early 1970's, Wyeth Laboratories withdrew its vaccine from the marketplace. By the end of 1976, Pfizer stopped manufacturing vaccine for sale in the United States. From the latter part of 1977 until the end of 1999, only Lederle has manufactured this product for the United States market. In the year 2000, the Centers for Disease Control no longer recommended the use of Oral Polio Vaccine in the United States.)

The shame of all this is the fact that homeopathic immunizations formulas called nosodes, have been available for all illnesses and used effectively by thousands. These homeopathic remedies can be made from live virus pustules and thus convey real immunity to the actual human virus used as opposed to Western medical immunizations which sometimes use sterilized viruses which alters the DNA and behavior of a virus initiating not yet fully understood immune reactions. Still many mothers are understandably intimidated by a doctors who recommend some or all of these injections and other mothers are just afraid and do not do the research or have the courage to stand up for their baby's health and reject the establishment's advise. I always give my patients' vaccine waivers (that the schools usually keep behind the counter and do not offer to parents unless one asks for it). These waivers the parents can sign by themselves in many states and the school has to legally accept them. However, in other states the parents have to get a clinician of oriental medicine, chiropractic, homeopath, naturopath or Western medicine to sign these waivers saying that the child has received the immunizations.

As always, the more information one can receive and assimilate on the truth about various health issues, the better one can balance their intuition and intellect about health issues. However, when fear is present and one must go against the present mass-consciousness, many will not be able to make the courageous decision. For others, and I have known hundreds of them, it is perfectly natural not to give their babies injections or drugs of any type. Many healthy mothers with their intuitive capabilities still intact, understand the lack of need for a Western drug orientated baby doctor. Babies (and adults) naturally draw bacteria and viruses to themselves to strengthen and clean their bodies and these so-called colds and illnesses will usually stop by themselves if the baby and mother are on a healthy raw diet.

NURTURING A TODDLER'S INSTINCTIVE SURVIVAL /RAWDIET TO ENGENDER AN ENERGETIC CONNECTION TO THE SOURCE

The baby will naturally learn one of two things as it grows: that it can rely on its own energy and etheric/subtle body strength to heal itself as it grows and does not need toxic drugs or that it is too weak and impotent, needs toxic drugs and submits to the parents worry and anxiety. Fortunately, many children will intuitively reject their parents erroneous decisions by resisting being fed drugs and may even vomit afterwards in a primitive, wise and instinctive reaction to being poisoned. Some parents will, upon seeing such a strong resistance, intuit that this is not what the child needs and respect the child's instinctive wisdom and thus, foster the child's senses, instincts and later intuition about many of life's issues. Most parents, unfortunately, will just forcibly feed the drugs to their child and miss out on a great life lesson and path.

DIETARY ENERGIES

One can teach the child diet in 2 different ways initially divergent but eventually parallel directions. If one is able to provide those foods that are scientifically designed by various methods for kids there can be benefit. One can work with this by understanding as much as possible about the previous generations i.e., grand-parents etc. If the parents had one main eating habit for their whole life you should go back two generations. If parents had made significant shifts you can work with just that generation or one before if the natural diet shifts occurred about ten years before conception of the child. Data collected as to what will be passed on in terms of tendencies with regard to toxic materials, heated fats (lipid oxides), cooked proteins(heterocyclic amines), cooked carbs(acrylamides), plasticizers(phthalates), enzyme deficiencies etc.. . Mom plays a larger role than dad but you can see as kids actions tend to be more like one parent than the other.

Intuitive awareness can be nurtured by various means and analysis of palm, iris, and skin-tone. As the body reflects what is happening at the inner level at the outer level. Sometimes this backfires and this pushes changes ahead too much than is appropriate for the child's karma. In intuitive development one focuses as clearly as possible at developing the intuitive understanding that the child awakens. The critical time is around 7 years of age when the etheric higher consciousness separation from the parents happens and the teeth come in. If habits created with regard to intuition are those which are clearly a part of the eating process the child will take this for life. This is rarely emphasized and understood except in instinctives who are working with instincts at a family level. Some of the dietary methodologies instincts are present at birth but they get stronger as the child ages beginning at a level of observable intensity around 1-2 years old.

It is important to expose the toddler to a variety of well-known healthy foods in various conditions to foster the child's natural ability to observe what is happening in the physical body.

At 1-3 years old there will be much focalization on immediacy as one does does not have a good sense-of -time and this is ok, but the child will respond more to taste and immediate sensation in the physical body. Later, after-effects will be more conscious-5 minutes, then 10 minutes etc.. after eating. These important effects will build a reservoir of instinctive reaction and understanding within the child. In that sense parallel development by both scientific and instinctive means is valuable. You will recognize that simply correcting nutritional deficiencies brought on by generations by immediate contamination or difficulties etc.., is not the whole answer.

Parents are there to teach and educate so that the soul is touched by which the individual is able to make a significant leap in consciousness or understanding during the intermissive period or next life i.e. evolution.

So when you eat a food, it makes sense to ask how do I feel inside my body. Take a moment to do this in the presence of the child; within a few feet of the child there is a natural transfer so the child will then more easily be able to receive this way of receiving information so when he eats, a similar pattern is established and he will more consciously receive what this food is doing to the body.

How does it feel in my stomach , my esophagus, my taste buds. As it enters my blood , what is the unique sensation and energies and associations with the past, present and future. You see this so obviously with habit patterns established over and over between parents and kids with regards to eating foods, yet little understood as to how this can be established at a positive helpful level not an override of one's own primitive ideals but encouraging increasing of the instinctive reaction to food. This is critical when the child enters the teen years (the astral body integration, i.e., hormonal shift) and is so widely exposed to peer pressure generated by those who have no intuitive awareness and instead have only been influenced by society and especially commercialism. So then the natural child can eat garbage fast food, process it out, and then naturally be drawn back to those foods that are more appropriate at that time. Scientifically, there is much benefit in eating the highest enzyme-rich food but one must also be connected to the instinctive awareness with a repertoire of choices made available.

Raw meat introduction into the diet is a very important aspect when the child needs such a shift or change, especially when cleansing is necessary as when high levels of saturated cooked fats, various chemicals, and other aspects of contamination are trapped in the body, meat can be a powerful way of strengthening. However, meat wouldn't be necessary if the child can have sufficient nutrition by various other means in particular a variety of raw food and vegetables, sufficient dairy fats or coconut fat, oils, and others. **The body has a remarkable ability at a young age to develop enzymes necessary and digestive properties to work with what is available.**

But raw meat is an obvious advantage as it is the exact chemical balance of the materials used to produce the body's raw meat musculature and organs.

Gestation occurs for many years and a child's ability to work with many of the subtle energies and be able to understand them is just as important as the scientific aspects. Make taste as connected to nature as possible as in picking herbs for a sauce so one understands the inherent connection between nature and taste. Finding these ways of building these understandings is important because the child wants understanding , consciousness- where does this food come from?

This is the other aspect with respect to intuition that is so strongly discouraged when you provide a food already fully processed as in the typical fast food hamburger- it is so far removed from anything that can be imagined with regards to nature that there is no intuitive understanding of inherent energies. Becoming more aware of these energies is a powerful means for a child to be able to make the leap forward to be exposed to this evolution this lifetime: the understanding that the direct energy that nurtures and develops the plant and animal is that which can directly nurture and develop humans. Sunlight, water energy, and soil energy have as their developmental energies that which are primordial based on the physics of the sun and here the inert gases are truly revolutionary in human evolution and healing. It is therefore not just a matter of seeing at a knowledge level the transfer of energy from nature into food into the human body but **understanding that the basic energy of the universe as manifested in the sun's physics is that which provides manifestation of physicality !**

References

1. Lecture by Dr. Spencer Wells on his new book called on 11-03
"The Journey of Man: A Genetic Oddysey" which traces
the present human species origin, via the chromosome lin
eage, back to Africa only 60,000 years ago which is sur
prisingly recent, and shows how we are all, in a genealogi
cal sense, African in origin.

2. Vaccinations- The Silent Killer, A Clear and Present Danger.

Ida Honorof and E. McBean, Ph. D, N.D., P.O. Box 5449,
Sherman Oaks, CA. 91403 (1977).

3. Smallpox Vaccine and Aids .Pierce W. London Times, May 11, 1987.

4. Sugita et al *Acupuncture regulates leukocytes in human
peripheral blood.* Oxfd Journ. 2006;4:447-453

5. Tsura H. et al *Acupuncture on the blood flow of various organs*
Meiji University 2004

6. Wagner B. et al *effect of acupuncture on neutrophil respiratory
Burst.* Complem. Ther. Med 2003;11:4-10

7. Hisamatsu T. et al *Acupuncture stimulation enhances splenic
NKC cytotoxicity.* Showa Univ, School of Med 2003

Vibrational Treatments

Dr Samuel Hahnemann—(1755-1843) was the German physician who founded and brought homeopathy to prominence. He is the modern founder of homeopathy which in part, and to oversimplify, is a system which undertakes to cure a disease by means of a greatly diluted form of the agent which causes the disease. Homeopathy promotes the idea that "miasms" are the root cause of all chronic disease. **Miasms are seen as the vibrational root of most inherited diseases in the body.** Miasms often involve microorganisms like viruses and bacteria which may lie latent in cells for years as immunology now has proven with many common viruses. A growing per-cent of cancer is also now thought to be caused by viruses. Sometimes these microorganisms express themselves or become active causing illness or other imbalances for which a diagnose or cause is difficult. The same miasm may manifest differently in different people. While one's grandfather may have had the TB miasm manifesting in classical TB, the same miasm may display itself as asthma in the son or grandchild. Homeopathic remedies made from the offending agent can potentially clear miasms, as well as the toxin to which one was exposed, from both the cellular structure and the subtle bodies. **Nosodes** are homeopathic remedies that are made from diseased tissues. So it is made from a minute sample of tissue affected with the bacteria. The sample may also be diluted to such a degree that there is no detectable physical evidence of the original agent. The miasms are generalized into the following groups each of which manifest in unique patterns in human chakras, organs and subtle bodies: **Psora, Tubercular, Syphilitic, Sycotic, Cancer, Petrochemical, Heavy Metal, and Radiation.** Again the miasm theory is mentioned here to entice readers to research it themselves. **Miasma are a genetic predisposition to a disease but they are also a great energy source** to thrive and evolve.

As humans age, their vitality or life force ("chi" or "ki' or "prana") weakens which allow miasms to manifest in the physical body. They may be seen as a crystallized form of karma. **Miasms are not the disease** but the potential for disease. The lack of chi/ ki and raised consciousness could be seen as the miasm. When the ki/chi is strong and consciousness is raised, the life force penetrates into the miasm and it does not produce illness. (Miasms may also be stored outside the physical body in the subtle bodies eg., etheric, astral, and causal. The solid human body is considered as a lower frequency replication of some aspects of the subtle bodies which help form it. The so-called **7-rays** mediate aspects of the subtle bodies-chakras interconnection.) **A strong psycho-spiritual orientation is thought to potentially obviate the miasms' manifestation of disease and its intended lessons.**

I am only mentioning homeopathy-like healing as it is so complex and powerful one needs to read the literature available. Hopefully readers will look into this, research it, and try it for the deepest healing. Personal clinical experience has demonstrated to me that vibrational treatments are often very comprehensive and effective. **Homeopathy, flower essences, gem elixirs and other such treatments seem to affect the patient on many subtle energy levels** that, while the patient may or may not acknowledge these, may well initiate healing cycles in the subtle bodies that eventually manifest in either the body physical or emotional.

The way that vibrational remedies are thought to work is fascinating and I will summarize some theories. Different forms of what are known as vibrational remedies, if ingested, **enter the meridians after resting between the circulatory and nervous system. An electromagnetic current is created by the polarity of these two systems.** Steiner and Blavatsky spoke of a connection between these two systems in relation to the life force and consciousness. The meridians may use this passage between the nervous and circulatory system to support the life force in the body physical. **The meridians may be the interface between the properties of the ethereal and physical bodies.** Such theories support the role of acupuncture in promoting human health at various levels. From the meridians, the vibrational remedies life force may enter the various subtle bodies (etheric, astral, causal etc), the chakras, or returns to the physi-cal body via various portals like the chakras or skin. Toxins are thought to be pushed out to the edge of the outer aura for purification. **Some toxins are probably pushed into the ethers where they are purified while the human mind pulls many toxins back into the body physical.** As mentioned earlier, most remedies and healings only temporarily balance the energies to allow for a readjustment of consciousness and a release of emotional attachments and misconceptions.

Some remedies seem to align with what in metaphysics is called the "higher dimensions" establishing a gentle resonance, which gets started, and increases over time to attunement to higher subtle energies of the patient. A specific connection to Mother Earth as the 8-12 Hz (Schumann resonance) is more easily established. The Schumann resonance is also known in Buddhism as the Earth's heartbeat and averages the same frequency as the human brain's alpha wave. Technically, the Schumann resonances are quasi-standing electromagnetic waves that exist between the surface of the Earth and the inner edge of the ionosphere 55 kilometers up. The standing waves represent several frequencies with the fundamental one being 7.8 Hz. (HansVolland,1995).

There are many ways in which the human body, plants, animals and minerals have changed since evolution began which necessitate a fresh new perspective on biology and acupuncture theory as taught in schools today. It was interesting to see how little the energetic and biology theories and textbooks had changed between when I finished Oriental Medical School in 1990 and when my twin sister went to Oriental Medical School in 2002

What I feel is interesting to consider is the way in which an individual may have been exposed to various healing techniques or pain in this life or a past life. For example, many people have in-teresting reactions to "moxa" (*artemesia* vulgaris). **Moxa** is a plant commonly used to warm or cauterize different acupuncture points on the body. These reactions relate to breathing the fumes and the various particulate matter. Some of these were not present in past times because the herb itself has changed has had all DNA from eons past. **Each human generation sees approximately thirty new genetic mutations from each parent** (lecture by MIT researcher Eric Lander 2002) but most of these are not on genes. Background radiation is the main agent of mutation over eons.[A 11-2003 lecture by Dr. Spencer Wells on his book called, "The Journey of Man: A Genetic Oddysey" which traces the present human species origin, via the mitochondrial DNA lineage (inherited only from the female as the mitochondria passed on all come from the female cytoplasm) back to Africa only 60,000 years ago which is more recent than previously theorized!]

In many cases moxa and other plants have been contaminated with various toxic materials from the atmosphere, aluminum in particular, which is not a good thing for anyone to be breathing. We already have so much heavy metal toxicity accumulated in our bodies from the food we eat and air we breathe. However, one can receive some positive effect from moxa, because one is tuning into past life energies associated with the herb, the treatment, the warmth and other matters.

When placement of moxa is accurate i.e., on the acupuncture point and not just near it, there is a direct relationship to the body being able to absorb and work with the fiery warming energy that, empirically, many people find tonifying and comforting.. I prefer lasers and various electronic technologies over moxa to directly impart energies into the meridians because it avoids risking the various pollutants. However, I have found that one can still bridge past-life attunement with the essential oil of mugwort or in other ways.

[Another form of this *artemesian* plant has been used effectively for centuries for fever, malaria and cholera-like diseases in S.E. Asia. The World Health Organization has been recommending it widely as a malarial treatment since 2001. As malaria has increased its resistance to conventional anti-malarial drugs like chloroquine, sulfadoxine-pyrimethamine and amodiaquine, Artemisinin-based combination therapy proved more effective and have been recommended in all countries where falciparum malaria (the most resistant form) is endemic. Artemisinin has been proven to be effective in treating all types of malaria including Plasmodium falciparum in areas with a high rate of resistance against other antimalarials. In African countries, artemisinin derivatives showed the same efficacy. The sesquiterpen-lacton-peroxides in this plant act essentially as a blood schizontocide. (McIntosh HM, Olliaro P. Artemisinin derivatives for treating uncomplicated malaria: *The Cochrane Library*,2002)(I and many of my friends used hydroxychloroquine in SE Asia in the 1990s for malaria. It was just 2 doses and made all of us feel sick. It has an incredibly long half-life of 50 days so a very little will still be in your body after a year)

Healing therapies can provide a time to heal and attune to the sacred healing earth frequency. This Schumann frequency has always been considered one of healing within metaphysics and most native cultures. All we have to do is be conscious of it and attune to it over time. It is always present everywhere we walk and sleep daily yet few consciously take advantage or are even aware of this energy bestowed upon all of us. This can be a two-way communication.

However, **for some people any frequency or subtle energy technique will be insufficient for healing because they need more physicalized treatment that cannot be brought by subtle energy** alone. Hence, the necessity and advantage of a healing raw food diet. Usually a raw food diet high in raw fats is necessary before one can fully benefit from many acupuncture treatments because the treatments are too strong a stimulus for an impaired nervous system that most people suffer from. **As nerves are high in various lipids, most people's nerves (hence brain) have been starving for decades.**

"Can You Adjust My Frequencies?"

Many frequencies that relate to all health relate to DNA frequency oscillation movement change and the interrelationship between the helixes themselves. These heli have various and subtle yet complex frequency interactions which must typically extend into the megahertz range. Therefore, when a patient asks about frequency adjustment, as many do, I appreciate the question.

However, such a question is too vague since the body is far too complex when it comes to frequencies. High frequencies can be adjusted by various structures but the capacity to modulate or shift such energies does come from the consciousness of the person. Therefore, I usually try to coach the patient and explain the basic physics and metaphysics behind the science of geometric biological formations, electric/magnetic/crystal combinations and other subtle energies as best I can.

Applying frequencies to a 7-foot by 7-foot copper, crystal, and gold pyramid as I work has proven interesting over the years. **Certain electrical units utilize waveforms that mimic the specific type of waves as found in the acupuncture meridians.** Other wave forms applied externally allow one to form complex wave forms utilizing simple division of frequency theories so frequencies are brought into the brain wave region and many **specific interrelationships between frequencies in the human brain region and human voice frequency have been discovered yet the ultimate wave forms themselves remain as sine waves.**

T.E.N.S. (transcutaneous electrical nerve stimulation) units and certain wave forms will at times produce some higher har-monics that the patient will find disturbing and are not desirable (nausea, vomiting and insomnia). Overriding the galvanic currents in the pyramid itself was in the end not so difficult as a simple T.E.N.S. unit was sufficient. Certain electrical units attached to a magnetic/copper mat in various geometric designs can make a nice coupling to the spine. However, after many years I finally saw that the use of magnetic fields that permeate the physical body have a far greater capacity to engender this resonant response. Electrical stimulation does cause nerves to fire, but this is too stressful or people's impaired nervous system today as their diets lack sufficient raw fats. Direct magnetic stimulus has proved thus far the most effective and least stressful for most people. **The brain has the highest number of neurons and is thus most susceptible to magnetic field interaction.** Utilizing a number of frequencies has been used in all kinds of research for the communication of specific tones and colors. Yet, if these carrier waves have impressed upon them powerful healing aspects by an experienced healer this also will be transmitted.

Patients often do not realize that every type of body part has a frequency associated with it at which that gland, organ or muscle functions most efficiently. When an ideal frequency is established as, for example, through voice tones, these tones can then be used as a sort of tuning fork to help adjust the sick organ's frequency. The usual published body part frequencies usually relate to measurable specific audio frequencies. In looking at the frequency of organs, you are also looking at a much higher frequency connection related to DNA associated with that part of the body that apparently will typically extend into the megahertz range.

The best way to measure these will probably be "in-vivo" and the human being presents many complex frequencies one on top of the other so it is difficult at times to isolate any single frequency. **DNA seems to have some coiling and uncoiling action that is constantly allowing an oscillatory motion and this would be more easily measured in the liquid environment; thus, blood DNA may be a bit easier to measure than the more solid DNA of denser material.**

The interesting thing is that there is a direct octave frequency relationship and this frequency must be borne by the brain. The brain itself must be able to shift these frequencies and work with them all the way to macro-brain patterns that occur across the entire brain and are those that are easily picked up by e.e.g. (electro-encephalograph). **Hence, providing frequencies associated with an organ can allow the brain to move into a condition of a sense of equilibrium or even entrainment.** This can be particularly helpful if octave relationship is applied so that you lower the frequencies until you come to the 7-21 cps brain wave patterns.

Now, buried within the human voice is the reflex pattern you will see in the other body parts such as the ear and eye that are well known. This reflex pattern is also established within the potentially sacred human voice, but insufficient voice analysis techniques are available to understand this completely. **Thus the important emphasis of many on developing the throat area chakras.** However, there are those that study and work with this and have come up with sounds that are very healing. Similarly, there are some people who sing, chant, or bring sounds that are inherently very healing to the human body, and this is where the use of frequency to name these sounds is really appropriate, is measurable and that with which people in their singing are able to work. **As a result, in many ways it is the most accurate way of working with the frequencies of an organ.** (I remember many healing sessions listening to the monks chanting). I suspect that the voice healing will eventually be a far better tuned, more accurate way of healing with frequency than would be anything of pure instrumentation or technology.

In metaphysical literature, the human body is usually divided into 7-12 subtle "layers" of a more etheric nature that lie outside of our physical body. Some find it easier to visualize these layers to octaves on a piano as **each octave has a higher frequency yet each octave shares a sympathetic resonance as in harmonics.** The first layer is called the **etheric body that "builds" as well as imbues the physical body.** These subtle bodies relate to how we receive energy from the higher aspects of our soul and spirit. The seven main "chakras" are energy portals that connect/transform higher energies from our subtle bodies into our seven endocrine glands and then our physical body.

Steiner writes that the Ancients held that the fluids of the human body carried into the organism forces derived from the cosmos itself. Such cosmic forces were regarded less and less as the centuries went on; but nevertheless medical thought was built up on the remains of the fading conceptions of Hippocrates until the fifteenth century. Contemporary scientists therefore have great difficulty in understanding pre-fifteenth century treatises on medical subjects; and we must admit that the writers of these treatises did not, as a rule, themselves fully comprehend what they wrote. They talked of the four elements of the human organism, but their special description of these elements was derived from a body of wisdom that had really perished with Hippocrates. Nevertheless, the qualities of these fluids were still matters of discussion and dispute. In fact, from the time of Galen till the fifteenth century, we find a collection of inherited maxims that become continuously less and less intelligible. Yet there were always isolated individuals able to perceive that there was something beyond what could be physically or chemically verified, or included in the merely terrestrial. Such individuals were opponents of what "humoral pathology" had become in current thought and practice. And chief among them were Paracelsus and Van Helmont, who lived and worked from the end of the fifteenth century into the seventeenth, and contributed something new to medical thought, by their attempts to formulate something their contemporaries no longer troubled to define. But the formulation they gave could only be fully understood with some remainder of clairvoyance, which Paracelsus and Van Helmont certainly possessed. **If we ignore these facts, we cannot arrive at any conclusion concerning peculiarities of medical terminology whose origin is no longer recognizable.**

Paracelsus assumed the existence of the Archaeus, as the foundation for the activity of the organic "humours" in man; and his followers accepted it. He assumed the Archaeus, as we today speak of the "Etheric" body man.

Whether we use the term Archaeus, as Paracelsus did, or our term, the etheric body, we refer to an entity which exists but whose origin we do not trace. If we were to do this, our argument would be as follows: **Man possesses a physical organism mainly constructed by forces acting out of the sphere of the earth; and also an etheric organism mainly constructed by forces acting from the cosmic periphery.** Our physical body is a portion as it were of the whole organism of our Earth. Our etheric body—like the Archaeus of Paracelsus—is a portion of that which does not belong to the earth, but which acts on and affects the earth from all parts of the cosmos. Thus Paracelsus viewed what formerly designated the cosmic element in man—of which the knowledge had perished with Hippocratic medicine—in the form of an etheric body, which is the basis of the physical. But he did not investigate further—though he gave some hints—the extra-terrestrial forces associated with the Archaeus and acting in it.

The exact significance of such facts grew more and more obscure, especially with the advent of Stahl's medical school in the seventeenth and eighteenth centuries. Stahl's school has wholly ceased to comprehend this working of cosmic forces into terrestrial occurrences; it grasps instead at vague concepts such as "vital force" and "spirits of life." Paracelsus and Van Helmont were con-sciously aware of the reality at work between the soul and spirit of man and his physical organisation. Stahl and his followers talk as though the conscious soul-element was at work, though in another form, upon the structure of man's body. This naturally provoked a vehement reaction. For if one proceeds like this and founds a sort of hypothetic vitalism one comes to purely arbitrary assertions, and the nineteenth century opposed these assertions. Only a very great mind, like Johannes Müller (the teacher of Ernst Haeckel), who died in 1858, was able to overcome the noxious effects of this confusion, a confusion of soul forces with "vital forces" which were supposed to work in the human organism, although how they operated was not very clear.

Meanwhile a quite new current made its appearance. We have followed up the other current which faded out; the new current in the nineteenth century had a rather different bearing upon medical thought. It was set in motion by one extremely influential piece of work dating from the preceding century: the *De sedibus et causis morborum per anatomen indugatis* by Morgagni. Morgagni was a physician of Padua, who introduced an essentially materialistic trend into medicine; the term materialism is used here, of course, as an objective description, without sympathies and antipathies. The new trend initiated by Morgagni's work consisted in turning the interest to the after-effect of disease upon the organism. Post-mortem dissections were regarded as decisive; they revealed that whatever the disease may have been, typical effects could be studied in certain organs, and the changes of the organs by disease were studied from the autopsy. With Morgagni, pathological anatomy begins, whereas the former content of medicine still retained some traces of the ancient element of clairvoyance. (Refer to Dr. Rudolph Steiner's <u>Anthroposophical Approach to Medicine</u> Anthroposophical Press. 1957. **Chakras are considered to be energy vortexes in our subtle bodies that connect with the physical body and adjust higher vibrational energies.** There are seven main chakras that relate to our seven main endocrine glands and their related organs. Overall, there are 360 chakras. See also Alice Bailey, <u>Esoteric Healing</u> N.Y. Lucis Publishing Co., 1980.)

There are well-known subtler type (higher vibrational) energies around all people that I have learned can be potentized and even directed with various subtle energy technologies (such as inert gases, lasers, certain geometric structures made from certain materials, crystals etc...) in the treatment room. These augmented and purified energies actually make the acupuncture more successful because there is more energy involved. Unfortunately, there is a serious downside to this when acupuncture is utilized without protective subtle technologies in an environment of rather high levels of etheric congestion such as Tokyo, New York City and especially Hong Kong. In a crowded treatment setting, there can be some difficulty as most people have subconsciously developed increased sensitivity to the etheric energy coupled into the needles. The puncturing itself causes energetic shifts and this is the main topic of both teaching and research in modern acupuncture schools and hospitals. **However, what is not considered by most people is that the needles allow for an attunement to both the higher vibrational and etheric energies around a person at the time** of needling and it is this that causes benefit and assistance. It is also this surrounding energy that is of more profound importance as time goes on.

This etheric "congestion" also helps explain the benefit of having needles inserted into one's body in a "protected" environment, which shields one from others' interfering energies. There are many ways to prevent people's energies from mixing inappropriately but I have found that a properly designed appropriate geometric structure such as a pyramid (made from material such as gold, copper, crystals and magnets) the most simple and effective to use. Many of my patients also really prefer treatments inside a beautiful powerful pyramid.

I often saw odd effects on patients in Tokyo or Hong Kong, which I thought were just emotional problems and quirks that one often sees in large crowded Asian cities. Later, I concluded that these effects were usually just short-term emotional imbalances brought on by the patients' needles acting as antennae transmitting confusing thoughts and energies from the surrounding people directly into them. Some individuals do not respond positively to placement of needles in some points. The healer is required to intuit why the patient is reacting to various techniques and point stimulus. These reactions vary from many different physical sensations to emotional outbreaks, commonly crying or sadness or considerable shaking. I always hold the patients hand and reassure them that what they are feeling is normal and that it will subside soon. If necessary, I will adjust the needles or lasers to stop the reaction if it is too strong. These emotions can be used to help further diagnose the patient.

References
Abe, K. Hamasaki, K. Kojima, M. Sasaki, Jpn. J. Appl. Phy(1994)   Gurudas. Gem Elixirs and Vibrational Healing Casandra Press 1989 Hunt, Valerie. Infinite Mind: The Science of Human Vibrations 1989 Volland Hans Handbook of Atmospheric Electrodynamics,1995

Microbes (virus, bacteria and parasites) evolved
way before humans to make us a perfect host for them in a
synergistic relationship. Any microbe that kills quickly as in HIV,
Ebola, SARS and MERS (two of 4 endemic corona viruses which
have a large genome) meaning we all have some natural immunity
to all corona strains) has logically been altered by humans for
various purposes. When a virus like the hemorrhagic Ebola
circulates, even a weakened form that we see now in Africa in 2017,
we will tragically see how this recent corona strain is comparatively
very mild. Ebola used to kill 100% of infected quickly so it couldn't
spread as much as everyone would die before they could spread it
from village to village. Now mutations have made it maybe only
50% fatal so it will be able to spread and could kill 100s of millions
as is. Ebola vaccines have failed and some limited medicines aren't
hopeful. Ebola is awful as it causes systemic internal bleeding.
Some viruses mutate too quickly for vaccines and anti-virals have
never worked well. **The human immune system has many
excellent antiviral capabilities!**

Another concern would be a virus manipulated to
detox humans of an organophosphate (herbicides like **glyphosate)**
as it is in all of us via our grains (breads, alcohol, contaminated
other crops). Very worrisome would also be a virus manipulated to
detox humans of fluoride as it is in all of us via city water and
therefore everything. **Fluoride** is small and not well filtered out.
**The only scientific way to prepare for coming pandemics is to
detox the body enough so that the microbe will have little
reaction in our body. However, all pandemics force us to work
together, help each other, empathize , prioritize and thus evolve!**

Low Deuterium Water (DDW)

In 2019, humanity was "blessed" by those who were inspired and seeded with the task of creating Low Deuterium Water (DDW- deuterium depleted water). It is available in the USA online now from 2 sources. Deuterium is a form if hydrogen (a heavy isotope of hydrogen. A deuteron is a fermion bound together with another fermion and is the atomic nucleus of deuterium). Earth's Deuterium comes from the sun naturally as the Earth ages more deuterium is deposited. This is the ultimate healing tool many have been waiting for. It had been an effective cancer therapy in animals in Europe. **Excess deuterium itself was well known to degrade the energy/ATP producing mitochondria in each cell -so less deuterium would logically help**. A brain neuron can have 1000s of mitochondria in them and the potential healing, slower aging, increased brain function and mental health from those neurons producing more happy neurotransmitters like serotonin and dopamine could be incredible. Mitochondria also have their own unique small DNA which can cause various illnesses. The mitochondria are passed on through the maternal line(actually the male mitochondria are destroyed by the egg cell after conception and the oocyte has the most mitochondria of any human cell--a hundred thousand!) . There is much online research available over the past decades.

I knew from research that present Earth water was generally 150ppm deuterium so food and body levels were about the same. Glacier water and animal fat measured lower like 100-130ppm.

I was able to buy the 25ppm 5 gallon jugs for 250us$. This was cheaper than the 25ppm or 50ppm bottles. I would dilute this with regular filtered water (which is always around 150ppm) to get 100ppm. After 12 weeks of 3 liters daily (diluted to 100ppm) water, I sent my saliva to an Australian lab I worked with (it cost only 75$ - much cheaper than the USA online saliva kits costing around 200$). Three weeks later I was happy to see my saliva was down to 110ppm from the starting point of 150ppm (which is average for most humans). However, the empirical data on DDW is recent, online, and from patients who were doing the DDW (deuterium depleted water) were the only evidence based information. It is very expensive so many patients refused to do it unless they were very ill, depressed, or dying. Understandable ! I lowered my dilution so instead of drinking 100ppm I started doing around 50ppm but I did start to drink less daily so now I was doing about 2 liters daily. Four months later I hit my goal of 80ppm. **Measuring deuterium levels is tricky as deuterium is an isotope of Hydrogen and is very small and its nucleus even smaller (as with tritium and protium) and test results fluctuate daily it seems looking at test results.** Therefore, the Heisenberg uncertainty principle applies i.e., the inquiry changes the results. Any measure of an excretory function, especially water based (hair, saliva etc) is best done at the same time of the day and month due to natural moon cycle changes. Also, using the same lab made sense for increased consistency.

One must remember to add up all other liquids and food to estimate daily intake. So if u drink regular water, coffee or a soda or eat food, meat etc remember those foods are counted at 150ppm. Still, like all effective therapies, even the DDW isn't healing 100% of the people I eventually contacted. Also, a couple people with high deuterium levels are also doing ok. **However, the healing of most with severe debilitating health issues is amazing and therefor DDW must be tried by as many as possible.**

The patient self-reports and clinical records will prove amazing over the coming years. **As low deuterium is such a logical scientific fundamental concept for healing most people should try it. It is logical that children raised on DDW will become a new longer living human. It has great potential for humans.**

Detox/Lymph Baths

The 105F , 90-minute detox baths take some effort.

Fortunately, most wouldn't do a cold bath but hot water is fine for most but too hot for some especially with different conditions. Still it takes time to fill up the tub, measure the water temp every 20 min once in and add more 130F water for 1 min to maintain at least 105F (I usually get in around 107.5F. Then it goes down soon because of human 99F body temperature). After about 30 min my body temp increases to 100 forehead reading. When I get out after 90 minutes of hot water and meditation, music etc the fever can be 101.5 on a digital thermometer (my base forehead reading with an infrared thermometer is 97.2 degrees so I add 1.6 degrees to the reading) so I became familiar with how it feels with a 103 temperature. It is disorientating and tiring and somehow very interesting. I would have to lie down and continue sweating a lot for an hour or three.

I knew that the hot blood/fever was key to healing and welcomed that disorientated feeling. Fevers force some toxins like food colorings and metals, to leave the brain and be expelled hopefully. Fevers can also break up certain toxins and cellular structures increasing antigen presentation so one's own immune cells, like T-cells could be triggered to detox certain elements and even cancer cells like some lymphoma cells.

The other main detox is that human fat melts at 105F and as that fat leaves the body it brings with it MANY stored toxins such as pthalates (plastics), acrylamides, heterocyclic amines, etc. This is also why gaining 20 pounds and taking it off helps detox so much- the toxins stored in the fat leave the body as one looses weight ! The bath seems more effective and easier for most- but why not do both!

Empirically, <u>fresh raw coconut cream and pineapple</u> **is the best scientific biochemical based lymph detox food I've seen** . Getting fresh cream from a coconut is an art and takes time and an expensive 350-700US$ slow speed 50-110rpm juicer warrantied for coconut (and no you cant use store bought not fresh pseudo coconut cream). It can be eaten daily as well as applied to the neck/axillary lymph node areas if you feel and see a swollen neck, throat, tonsils, or axillary glands and you can see your neck skin is red - these are some early common lymph problem signs and if chronic also seen in neck lymphoma (cancer). The pineapple, being high in enzymes etc , can sting and even burn if used on the skin too much -especially in the axillary. **It is great for acne also (applied topically)**. It will "dry" on the skin after 20 min or so and can be reapplied. The combination cream is yummy for most but can be a bit of a laxative so best to do a couple spoonfuls daily and build up to about 6-8 spoonfuls if you can. Especially before a detox bath is ideal.

The next important item is **raw organic white meat** i.e., fowl **because white meat is for the white blood cells (as raw read meat (beef bacon etc) is for the muscles and organs)**. Chicken or turkey breast is common. It is more popular to soak it in a baggie with lemon juice and some spice like ginger. This really makes it smell and taste nice as well as softening the meat. A little red meat for the magnesium seems to help maximize the chickens metabolism.

The final essential for lymph is **a <u>vibration machine</u>**(on amazon etc) which must be set at 5hz for lymph. Other frequencies have other advantages but 5Hz is empirically clearly most helpful with cancer patients. **10 min equals about 1 hour on a trampoline**. At least 1x a day minimum but 2-4x a day better. After 5 minutes you will get warmer and this also helps the lymph work better. You can stand or sit on it and put your hands flat down and feel it all over the body and especially in the upper back neck area.

Blueberries and raw cream seemed to be the best food detox for the brain and there is lots of good biochemical research online but the main point here is that some elements in blueberries have a good biochemical charge to magnetize various metals in the brain and drag them out of the brain. **But, as always one still has to get toxins out of the body physical !!!**

So many people have a great raw diet-high in animal fat and animal protein along with veggie juicing and raw dairy BUT they **never did enough real scientific detox so they never realized the maximum health and increased intelligence benefits of the diet as most of the toxins stayed in their bodies. Only the detox baths and 20lb weight gain-loss are scientifically physically effective and help ALOT. Many other things help a little but not much.**

Chi-kung moves done slowly to help the etheric para-brain (our physical organs have an etheric double in our etheric body). Elderly people especially see rapid improvement in coordination and memory. Any organ or gland can be worked on by doing these motions.

I had been using the **inert gas devices** which are, to my knowledge, the most advanced physical healing technology on Earth. These are various combinations or the inert gases (xenon, krypton, neon, helium and argon) pressurized and magnetized. Empirically, we use different gas % for different imbalances and for increasing certain capabilities, skills, meditations, etc. **These amazing gases seem to have the ability to heal the etheric body** (the subtle non-physical energy body double) and thus the physical. They seem to respond to thought forms about changing anything physically about one's body. **Intent is key. Usual thought forms and brain coherence is sloppy and weak like a dull flashlight. Intent and practice can make it more like a laser** (see pg 56). It seems that the physics behind it is based on the creation of physicality and life via the sun's helium gas energy.

As one realizes that the same direct energy that nurtures the plant and animal is that which can directly nurture humans. Sunlight, water energy, and soil energy have as their developmental energy that which are primordial based on the physics of the sun and here the inert gases are truly revolutionary in human evolution and development.

Therefore it is not just the knowledge of the transfer of energy from nature into food into humans but understanding the basic energy of the universe as manifested in the sun's physics is that which provides manifestation of physicality and here the inert gas potential is revolutionary yet, will never be used by most !!!

Tesla Coil and Scalar Wave Technology

This amazing new technology is scientifically not understood, but as always, using it with patients for just 2 years reflects wondrous potential that I will try to explain without the math and physics as I believe the reality to be. The math and physics are not known yet in Earth science but the ideas and words are very understandable to many now and it is some those ideas I will share. **Most people use these devices for brain entrainment but as you add/ connect different frequencies from any source (computer , phone, music or your own voice recordings saying "I love me" or "I am healthy/happy, " the potential is unlimited and evolving.) This is the highest frequency healing available commercially.**

By definition scalar is magnitude without direction but the physics definition falls short. Maxwell described scalar waves but he foolishly dismissed the scalar wave component in the solutions to the equations because it was seen as a spurious byproduct of the solution process being a term series of numbers and unknowns multiplied by the square root of negative one.

Scalar wave is produced by various means by which an interaction between a positive going and a negative going wave takes place like a caduceus coil (a wire is wound in one direction then the other direction so the same wire is carrying the same current allowing it to cancel). Cancellation is not perfect as there is always fringe effects at the edges of the coil. But at the centre of the coil there is no measurable magnetic field and yet this is where these actions that can be seen in a measurable way as in the UV spectrum of water- water exposed within such a coil has a shifted response to UV light. this can be stopped and repeated. Other methodologies also produce these energies. Using these energies with the inert gases is the next step. The math and science has not been developed yet but intuition and inspiration will show that the basic idea is that **the etheric energy normally present from any magnetic stimulation of inert gases has a higher frequency component with relationship to the human body when it is stimulated by a scalar wave. This can then be used to allow the causal body to interact with the other subtle bodies for great benefit.** Frequencies can be applied so that the inert gases allow for a series of harmonics that interact with human consciousness associated with the causal and atmic subtle bodies(discussed in the last chapter). Truly unlimited potential !!!

A good way to start the organic raw diet is to do what's easier. For most, that means veggie juicing, raw milk, and less cooked food each day. Just those 2 things can bring good changes and start to realign one's consciousness to the reality that all cooked food is carcinogenic and living in a state of unconscious starvation is not a way to be healthy and evolve.

As one start to feel better or different they often want to feel even better. Since raw animal fats increase some hormonal production, raw butter or cream usually **increases the libido** and for men the prostate fluid production.

If you want to improve the musculature and organs then raw meat will be best. Organic raw red meat like ground beef or bacon or the raw organs themselves are easiest for many and raw bacon actually tastes good and has always been a favorite with raw food people. One can add spices but I just eat it plain. Even one bite a day is enough to start changing energetic pathways. Likewise, organic raw white meat is fowl so chicken and turkey are common. Turkey tastes fine as is but chicken is preferred by most soaked in lemon juice and spice like ginger. The lemon juice makes chicken taste good and the texture also softens.

Just experimenting with some of these foods can be a life changer and open up your possibilities in life. One's soul often waits a lifetime for one to show some self love and respect by eating non-toxic food. **Have fun with it !**

I was taught by my Kagyu teachers that animals have decided on a group soul level, in a last desperate attempt, to offer themselves up to humans hoping that humans will acquire some of the animal understanding and and instincts and realign with nature so that humans stop destroying Mother Earth.

DIETARY BASICS

Carcinogens and mutagens are produced by highly heating food-meat, fat, grains etc (see intro and pg 82)

Enzymes are ruined my very low heat(average 115F)

Resins in cooked vegetables are toxic and aren't excreted

The **Brain** is 60% dry weight fat and half of that is animal fat

Pesticides and **herbicides** are on grains, fruits and vegetables (90% of breads, cereals, and alcohol contain **glyphosate**)

Microbes are designed to clean human bodies of toxins

Bacteria produce happy chemicals like Serotonin & Dopamine. Studies show low bacteria = brain problems !

Human DNA includes a lot of viral, bacterial and parasitical DNA

Therefore eating organic raw: meat, dairy, fruits,veggies, fats and ingesting 1000s of bacterial strains will produce a happy healthy human. The brain especially needs a lot of animal fat to allow for ideal function and happy mental health neurotransmitters.

Basic Nature Healing

One must **not forget or dismiss the origin and healing source energy for all life being the elements in the stars, Mother Earth, and our star, the Sun.**

We are all composed of elements on the periodic table which originated in stars and brought to the Earth by various means. Understanding human non-earth origin puts things in perspective. Allowing healing directly by being in the Sun and standing barefoot in the Earth will alway be one of the easiest most healing things to do. **Morning Sun before 1030am has little of the blue light spectrum which is so damaging to humans.** Blue spectrum from any source (computers, LED, sunlight) **damages human mitochondria** and must be reduced as much as possible.

Morning Sunlight is particularly healing in other ways because the Sun's etheric body is healing to all etheric bodies of Earthlings. Gazing directly at the 1st earliest morning Sun for a few minutes has special healing properties and of course is perfectly safe due to the minimal radiation at sunrise. Sun gazing is an ancient basic practice as is early morning sun bathing. Some Sun benefits, like Vitamin D3 production (vitamin D regulates 100s of genes), need a lot of skin surface so nude is best but the least clothing the better. 20 minute exposure and no water on skin for 45 minutes beforc AND after is required. Longer morning Sun exposure is needed to repair skin damage and some lymph based issues.

If sun bathing is done while sitting or lying on the grass or sand, it is the best healing spa. **The Earth energy, the Schumann resonance, and all the Earth's minerals, plants, microbes, soil, and especially the dominant quartz crystal content make the Earth the largest strongest source of various energies for all life on Earth.**

Reality over Illusion

It is important to remember that what was expressed on page 173 in bold print- (The baby will naturally learn one of two things as it grows: that it can rely on its own energy and etheric/subtle body strength to heal itself as it grows and does not need toxic drugs or that it is too weak and impotent, needs toxic drugs and submits to the parents worry and anxiety)- has huge implications for the life of any individual.

I always tell my patients (and my own children)that anyone can, in theory, heal themselves in various ways (or for minor complaints just wait and the problem will resolve itself) but by taking a pill or doing other therapy the main complaint often goes away more quickly and makes one more comfortable. However, often times when one does not heal themselves they are undermining their inherent healing connection to their non-physical energy source. My feeling is that the soul would love for us to acknowledge and feed on this energy source eventually so we don't have to wait till the next reincarnation.

Even just common over the counter pain or allergy medicine or any cooked food weakens us each time we ingest them, day after day, as though the inherent energy connection gets thinner and thinner till it can barely transmit energy at all and we are left impotent and dependent on non-self remedies- our consciousness barely able to even consider self-healing.

All it takes is to acknowledge our inherent life source and decide not to take that pill or eat that cooked food today and the source energy thread begins to heal! It is so basic and so powerful yet so hard as we are indoctrinated and literally brain-washed from childhood by our parents, society and the media. As humans now living on Earth, where we are so fortunate to now be able to easily access so much information, we must look behind this perverted ridiculous illusion and choose reality over the illusion.

AUTHOR

Paul Sweeney is a licensed acupuncturist also certified in pediatric mental health. He also has a background in microbiology. He has been doing martial arts and healing for 25 years including 10 years in Asia.

Being raised by parents who were both Western medical professionals, he was well aware of the pros and cons of Western medicine. His mother also introduced him to both chiropractic and acupuncture from a young age and this was a wonderful influence by an intelligent open-minded mother. After finishing his undergraduate and graduate education in New England, he spent 10 years in various Asian clinics, dojo, hospitals and temples training and working with great teachers and healers of different styles trying to understand the nature of psychological and physical imbalances and how to address such. Paul now integrates raw diet, psychology, acupuncture, and martial arts with healing technologies discussed in this book.